Succeeding with Interventions
for Asperger Syndrome Adolescents

Succeeding with Interventions for Asperger Syndrome Adolescents

A Guide to Communication and Socialisation in Interaction Therapy

John Harpur, Maria Lawlor
and Michael Fitzgerald

Jessica Kingsley Publishers
London and Philadelphia

Information on Pragmatic Rating Scales on pp.74–5 is taken from 'Social Language Use in Parents of Autistic Individuals' by Landa, R., Piven, J., Wzorek, M.W., Gayle, J.O., Chase, G.A. and Folstein, S.E. (1992) In *Psychological Medicine 22*, 245–54. Reprinted with permission of Cambridge University Press.

Information on verbal and nonverbal discourse skills on pp.80–4 is taken from 'Enhancing Language and Communication Development: Language Approaches' by Prizant, B.M., Schuler, A.L. and Wetherby, A.M. (1997) In *Autism and Pervasive Developmental Disorders* edited by D.J. Cohen and F. Volkmar. New York: John Wiley & Sons, Inc. p.592. Copyright 1997 John Wiley & Sons, Inc. Reprinted with permission of John Wiley & Sons, Inc.

First published in 2006
by Jessica Kingsley Publishers
116 Pentonville Road
London N1 9JB, UK
and
400 Market Street, Suite 400
Philadelphia, PA 19106, USA

www.jkp.com

Library of Congress Cataloging in Publication Data
Harpur, John, 1958-
Succeeding with interventions for Asperger syndrome adolescents : a guide to communication and socialisation in interaction therapy / John Harpur, Maria Lawlor and Michael Fitzgerald.
   p. cm.
Includes bibliographical references and index.
ISBN-13: 978-1-84310-322-6 (pbk.)
ISBN-10: 1-84310-322-2 (pbk.)
 1. Asperger's syndrome--Patients--Rehabilitation. 2. Teenagers with mental disabilities--Rehabilitation. 3. Communicative disorders in adolescence--Treatment. 4. Interpersonal communication in adolescence. 5. Social interaction in adolescence. I. Lawlor, Maria, 1959- II. Fitzgerald, Michael, 1958- III. Title.
RJ506.A9H2685 2006
618.92'858832--dc22

2005035293

British Library Cataloguing in Publication Data
A CIP catalogue record for this book is available from the British Library

ISBN 978 1 84310 322 6

Printed and bound in Great Britain by
Athenaeum Press, Gateshead, Tyne and Wear

We dedicate this book to the many parents and professionals who strive to help adolescents with Asperger syndrome live happier lives.

Acknowledgements

The authors would like to acknowledge the many anonymous parents and adolescents with Asperger syndrome who helped to pilot the interaction skills intervention. Without their cooperation and dedication, the current work would not have reached fruition as quickly. Second, the staff and council of ASPIRE, the Asperger Syndrome Association of Ireland, have been unfailingly supportive of our efforts. In addition, the Health Research Board, Department of Health and Children, the National Lottery and Enterprise Ireland have funded various portions of the work reported here, either directly or indirectly. Particular thanks is due to Frances Fletcher of DHC. Third, a range of speech and language therapists, childcare therapists, and mental health professionals have given valuable insights into their daily practices, and the advantages and disadvantages of certain approaches to social skills training. Professor Rebecca Landa from Johns Hopkins gave two leading talks at a workshop which JH and ML organised in June 2004. The interaction was very helpful. We also compliment the wonderful staff at Jessica Kingsley Publishers whose dedication ensures the production of timely resources for all involved. In addition, there are those within our respective institutions, be they postgraduates or registrars, who have helped with materials and liaising with parents and adolescents. JH would particularly like to acknowledge three of his research assistants: Karen Ashton produced valuable work during the early stages of assessing the Pragmatic Rating Scale; Marjolein Deunk provided psychometric and data collection support; Linnea Bengtsson has collaborated in the analysis of adolescent conversation patterns.

Finally, we acknowledge that much of the success in research and writing happens because of the patience of families. We owe them a great deal of time back.

Contents

9   Evaluation Issues   191

Introduction

This book focuses on the development of *interaction skills* in adolescents with Asperger syndrome (AS) through teaching social competence. Its primary audience is the group of mental health professionals and teachers designing and delivering socialisation training to Asperger adolescents – the 'therapists' as we refer to them in the book. The term *socialisation* refers to a range of behaviours, emotions, judgements and skills that define and underwrite effective social communication and interaction. We use the term interaction skills deliberately since it identifies both the fundamental feature of all social contact, namely its interactive nature, and the fundamental *impairment* in Asperger syndrome. A large part of the book explains the necessary and satisfactory conditions for successful social interactions to occur. It is a bit of an academic mouthful admittedly, but we are dealing with complex and subtle forms of human expression and there is no merit in thinking otherwise. Any socialisation intervention, and any teacher of one, has to be mindful of these conditions. As a discipline, teaching social communication principles to AS adolescents is neither trivial to grasp or deliver.

By *adolescent*, we mean a child past puberty and under the age of 20 years. We signal clearly at the outset that a 'one size fits all' model is difficult if not impossible to achieve for those with AS. Differences in developmental stages coupled with the presence of other complicating conditions (e.g. depression, attention deficit hyperactivity disorder, obsessive compulsive disorder) will mean that a minority of adolescents need other therapies prior to and during any socialisation intervention. We think in terms of 'doing the most for the most'.

Parents will find value in the book, but they need to link its content to a group intervention for their adolescents and themselves. A large part of what we do resonates with what is termed social skills training (SST). We dislike the convenience of the phrase 'social skills' as it implies, perhaps unwittingly, that everyone except those with Asperger syndrome is socially skilled. The phrase *social competence* is preferable in our opinion, as it combines two strands in learning theory, the cognitive and the behavioural.

Another process emphasised in the intervention philosophy is *building social confidence*. Adolescents with Asperger syndrome often report lacking confidence when interacting with their peers. The absence of social confidence is acutely felt during adolescence more than at any previous time. Persuading the adolescent to think about social challenges differently, in terms of varying their understanding and solutions, is intrinsic to the cognitive restructuring that is necessary.

There is no doubt that school bullying of the AS adolescent exacerbates feelings of anger, anxiety, inadequacy and failure. Confidence building, alone and unsupported, is not sufficient to help the young person confront many everyday peer challenges. The intervention we elaborate here, a multimodal intervention, requires active parental involvement. Parents are the primary therapists in their everyday involvement with their children. They can help the young person capitalise an intervention by giving positive feedback on appropriate social behaviour, practising role plays, and creating opportunities for potentially successful peer contacts. We argue that any AS intervention must have parental modules to be effective.

In practice, we use video modelling quite extensively to assist with rehearsal, role play and feedback. Currently we have a bank of 56 videos covering 23 communication and interaction themes. In the text, we avoid referencing specific videos. For instance, we do not say 'Now play video X and ask the following questions'. Instead, we will refer to specific themes as required and describe the script model we use.

The attitudes of the therapist to the group and intervention delivery contribute mightily to the success of any intervention. The 'human' side of any therapeutic intervention is always complex. Outwardly uniform approaches may not produce uniform results. Experience and understanding play major roles, but a compassionate and empathic outlook must condition experience. Despite the volume of published work on Asperger syndrome and social skills, disproportionately little is directed towards developing therapists' attitudes and interpersonal delivery modalities. The increasing incidence of AS is putting pressure on a wider circle of agents than before. These agents (counsellors, parents, psychiatrists, psychologists, teachers and therapists) are expected to participate in and provide interventions without necessarily sharing the same understanding of autistic thinking. The impact of autistic thinking on the delivery of these interventions may be overlooked as a result. Resources and special education policies vary from place to place, and we make several suggestions in the book about how to best mange shortcomings.

Before embarking on an intervention as therapist, parent or participant, it is essential that one seek appropriate advice and guidance on any choice from competent professionals familiar with Asperger syndrome.

Finally, what does this book contain? Briefly, it describes the methodology, philosophy and science underpinning our approach to developing interaction skills in AS adolescents. It elaborates a template for an intervention that can be administered over six months to a year. There is sufficient information for professionals to add and subtract material while still holding fast to the underlying methodology. A full set of PowerPoint slides for use in the group intervention and the accompanying videos are available. For further details, please email: pragmatics@mindwareresearch.ie.

1 Background Issues in Social Skills Interventions

Background

Socialisation is a very compact term that refers to a whole bundle of processes by which a child learns to behave and integrate with peers and adults in socially acceptable ways. We take for granted that behaving socially entails the appropriate expression of speaking and listening skills, facial expressions and gesture movements, emotion control and display. For convenience, we categorise socialisation as having verbal, nonverbal and emotional components. Later in the chapter, we reclassify these further into cognitive, behavioural and emotional components. The challenge laid down by socialisation, from a therapeutic perspective, is that almost everyone takes it for granted. Most people have satisfactory social interactions with others on a daily basis. Experience tells us that socialisation (like politeness) is not evenly distributed in society. Some people are very comfortable in social settings and may have proverbial buckets of confidence, while others occupy a middle ground that runs all the way back to people who do not interact with anyone.

Intervention programmes (or 'interventions') are tools in the therapist's hands. They are designed to change thinking, behaviour and emotion management in people where such processes are not being healthily expressed. An intervention is designed to 'intervene' and improve a person's functioning in some sphere. Interventions designed to improve social functioning are increasing at a phenomenal rate. This increase, fuelled largely by demand from the autism sector, is placing strains on existing mental health services. The range of specialists evolving to meet the demand for socialisation interventions is growing beyond traditional boundaries. What is more, intervention delivery and instructional methods themselves come under pressure during any rapid expansion of a service. This is especially true for interventions targeting adolescents on the autistic spectrum due to the scarcity of accessible interventions.

There is an insufficient number of skilled intervention therapists to meet the demand for services – most certainly too few to meet the demands of families. The transmission of knowledge, skills and attitudes to inexperienced professionals entering the field has become more pressing as time runs on. Currently only a few resources come even close to filling this gap. This book is an attempt to do so.

This chapter examines the process of 'bottling' socialisation interventions for adolescents with Asperger syndrome. Its focus on best practices will be of value to both experienced and inexperienced therapists. The chapter moves from a discussion of diagnostic issues on to the rationale for social skills training. This is then specialised for Asperger syndrome (AS), focusing on the adolescent. The chapter concludes with a review of various components for a broad intervention methodology.

Diagnostic issues in brief

Asperger syndrome (AS) is named after a Viennese paediatrician who noted that a number of his patients had pronounced communication and interaction difficulties (Asperger 1944). Over the past 25 years AS has been acknowledged as an autistic spectrum disorder characterised chiefly by impairments in social communication and interpersonal interaction. Despite the passage of time, the current scientific understanding of AS is incomplete. Existing research indicates that it is a neurodevelopmental condition, though the processes involved are incompletely understood. Speaking figuratively, the brain with AS is wired slightly differently from a typical brain.

The association of autism with Asperger syndrome has not always been readily accepted and therapists should take cognisance of that. There is a continuing debate as to whether high functioning autism is equivalent to having Asperger syndrome and vice versa (Klin, Volkmar and Sparrow 2000). Discriminating between the two categories, arguably, has little clinical significance especially in adolescence (Blacher et al. 2003; Frith 2004; Howlin 2003). Asperger syndrome is the preferred category in Europe for autistic people with normal intelligence, though the trend appears to be less established in the USA

(Mesibov *et al.* 2001; Schopler and Mesibov 1998). There are many excellent texts explaining AS from a variety of perspectives (developmental psychology, neuropsychiatry and autobiography) so the average reader is not distant from complementary sources of information (Attwood 1998; Gillberg 2002; Gillberg and Coleman 2000; Grandin 1996; Klin *et al.* 2000; Ozonoff and Miller 1996).

Irrespective of diagnostic debates, which are beyond resolution here, it is important to retain that often the apparent normality of those with AS in casual encounters can be entirely misleading. The social impairments, while organic, may be profoundly subtle. The significance of social impairments in the diagnostic criteria has weathered all clinical reappraisals of the criteria over the past 20 years. Interventions are an indispensable response.

Asperger syndrome is understood as a lifelong condition with its origins in prenatal development. No medical or pharmacological intervention exists that approximates to a 'cure'. Treatments may use pharmacology to manage co-occurring conditions and symptoms that interfere with a person relaxing and learning. These other conditions may include attention deficit hyperactivity disorder (ADHD), anxiety disorders, depression and obsessive compulsive disorder (OCD).

Positive features of AS may include perseverance in problem solving, passionate interest in an area of academic value and occasionally superior intelligence. Recent posthumous studies have uncovered inspirational role models for the AS adolescent to ponder upon. These figures are drawn from science, mathematics, music and literature (Fitzgerald 2004; Ledgin 2002). The majority of those with AS are unlikely to achieve these heights but many will have successful if less renowned careers (Baron-Cohen 2003).

Asperger syndrome is conveniently understood as autism with normal intelligence. This may not embrace all the clinical subtleties, but it is a workable definition. For over 30 years now, a triad of impairments has been accepted as defining the central autistic deficits (Wing and Gould 1979):

1. Impairments in imagination (e.g. inflexible cognitive orientations and processing).

2. Impairments in communication (e.g. failure to initiate conversation, inappropriate language, terse responses).

3. Impairments in social interaction (e.g. ignorance of nonverbal cues, abrupt or stiff body language).

A number of additional criteria separate the diagnosis of Asperger syndrome from severe autism, and chief amongst these are the normal to superior range of intelligence and intact verbal ability. Historically, Lorna Wing was probably the first to attempt a systematic analysis of Asperger's own criteria. She revised her triad of impairments criteria to include Asperger syndrome after having studied Asperger's own work (Wing 1981). Her revision includes reference to:

1. Impaired interpersonal communication.

2. General social clumsiness.

3. Poor repertoire of nonverbal communication behaviours.

4. Odd speech often coupled with pedantic forms of address and response.

5. Resistance to change.

6. Fondness for repetitive activities.

7. Selective intense interests (hobbies).

Wing's description of AS provided criteria that have been absorbed into widely used sets of clinical criteria. Where differences exist, they hinge on whether delayed early onset of language and motor clumsiness should be accepted into the criteria. For instance, the DSM-IV and ICD-10 both rule out early language delay, while other criteria admit it. It may seem like a side issue, but there is growing acceptance among mental health professionals that the criteria for Asperger syndrome need realignment. An informative review is found in Gillberg (2002). In what follows, the use of the Gillberg criteria is assumed unless explicitly stated to the contrary.

Reflection on diagnostic issues may seem premature, but clinical experience suggests that many parents are much less well informed on Asperger syndrome than can be divined upon meeting them. They usually require a 'cognitive walkthrough' of the criteria several times to grasp the implications of a diagnosis of Asperger syndrome for the child and family. A therapist should remind parents of the criteria when preparing to induct their daughter or son into an intervention.

Inexperienced professionals may be very impressed with some parents' knowledge of Asperger syndrome and its subtleties, only to have their expectations dashed when a parent fails to follow up on something 'obvious' to the professional. Exposure should not be confused with experience. Parents will have prolonged exposure to the condition, but they are rarely able to integrate their observations to the same degree as a professional with therapeutic experience and understanding of the condition. We go into more detail about parental involvement in AS-centred interventions in a later section.

Social skills training: the bewilderment factor

An intervention embraces more than training in social skills, but this is not self-evident. Discussing the therapy in terms of social skills training is often the best place to begin with parents, rather than introduce more theoretically intimidating concepts. More comprehensible is the idea that the intervention is about *social competence*. It captures notions of skill learning and good judgement (involving cognitive and emotional features). For the moment, however, we stick with the slightly narrower concept of social skills training.

The reaction of parents upon being advised that their child should attend some form of social skills intervention is often a mixture of dismay and bewilderment. While their dismay is profoundly private, their bewilderment at the need for social skills training is probably a common reaction. The bewilderment of many parents may go unnoticed with the risk that parental involvement in any intervention may be less effective.

From the outset, the structure of an intervention should be explained clearly to parents. Their questions must be answered. Parents will be naturally anxious about a change in routine for their adolescent. They may know from past episodes that he or she does not react well to change. Consent is required from both parents and adolescents. Consider this case study:

Mike was the father of a 16-year-old son with AS. His son had been out of school for almost a year. Mike was provided with all the documentation relating to the various assessment instruments that would be used in the study, a complete overview of the intervention's methods and aims, and a thorough explanation of the consent form. Despite having all the relevant information, Mike was still dissatisfied and thought he should receive more information and more time to reach his decision. *'I am just not clear about this'* or *'I am not sure about this here'* Mike would reply when asked if he understood the materials. Despite having the materials at home for several weeks, Mike was still unable to reach a decision (though his son wanted to participate). Eventually, the project leader told Mike in a calm tone that it was okay if he did not want to participate. He was entitled to withhold consent and the project team would not be the least offended. His anxiety was a reasonable response. The study would go ahead and perhaps he might participate in the future. Mike was quite surprised for a moment and then gave his consent.

Mike's reaction is very common. Many parents will have witnessed their children pass through a revolving door of all sorts of interventions and therapies with little measurable improvement in social interactions with peers. Many children with AS, especially in adolescence, have experienced a great deal of peer ridicule and rejection. Parents have shared in these misfortunes too. When another intervention is suggested, their first reaction is influenced by previous experiences of their child's failure and rejection in social settings.

Persuading parents to participate in an intervention needs careful thought. A percentage of parents experience having a child with a disability as a form of grief. The ideal child has been denied them. 'Why me?' 'What did I do wrong?' 'Why have I got such a raw deal?' are internal sentiments that parents may express from time to time. A therapist must be sensitive – not judge them. Parents may be depressed and have anxiety problems themselves. Having a child with a disability may place parental capacity for emotion regulation and psychological functioning under enormous strain resulting in marital disharmony and possibly breakdown.

Although these effects are partly visible to the therapist, extended family members and friends may not understand the implications of AS. They may behave in ways that parents find unsupportive. Parents may feel culpable for not being good parents, resulting in families with an AS child becoming more socially isolated from kin and friends.

Jean was diagnosed with Asperger syndrome at the age of 12 years. She was attached to a particular blanket and frequently refused to visit the homes of uncles and aunts unless she was permitted to 'wear' her blanket. A complicating factor was her dislike of certain fabrics used in underclothes. She also had a degree of motor clumsiness that resulted in occasional damage to domestic appliances, such as video recorders and DVD players. It emerged in family therapy sessions that friends and extended family members blamed the parents for Jean's behaviour. Their allegedly 'poor supervision' and 'lack of discipline' were topics for prolonged discussion at family occasions. Over a period of two years, Jean's parents withdrew from social outings, and the extended family dynamics deteriorated further. The arrival of Jean's family in family therapy arose largely from marriage guidance advice and the family doctor's concern with the mother's worsening anxiety disorder.

Emerging evidence suggests that there is a substantial genetic component to autistic spectrum disorders. It is probable, but not automatic, that a percentage of the parents will have pronounced AS traits. When this is the case, the affected parent is less likely to realise or understand the nature of the problems facing the adolescent. A parent may unintentionally minimise attendant difficulties. Crucially, they may also be less willing and less able to participate as the adolescent's guide, social agent and home-based therapist.

Parents will often remark that if training in something as obvious as social skills is required to help their son or daughter, there must be something terribly wrong. In fact, many people are looking for help with socials skills development. Browse any internet bookstore and there is a seemingly insatiable demand for social skills training in all forms. At the time of writing (summer 2005) a search of the internet using the phrase 'social skills' returned several million web pages across all categories. Refining the search with 'social skills autism' returned several hundred thousand pages. If further refinement is required then a search using 'social skills Asperger' returned tens of thousands of pages. There is a recognised global need across many sectors for social skills training. A vast plurality of approaches exists. With such choices available, bewilderment is inevitable – and it is certainly not limited to parents.

The fundamental puzzle of Asperger syndrome

The puzzle of Asperger syndrome lies in the following question: How can people of normal to superior intelligence, with good to excellent verbal ability, fail to learn even a small amount of the social conventions that infuse everyday human communication? Why are they failing to pick up the salient features of social interactions? A large number of studies indicate that AS people with notionally good verbal ability have a puzzlingly deficient comprehension of narrative, indirect discourse or figures of speech (Frith 1989; Happe 1993; Jolliffe and Baron-Cohen 1999; Jolliffe and Baron-Cohen 2001; Koning and Magill-Evans 2001). Paradoxically, they may be competent at analysing social problems that do not involve them directly (Baron-Cohen 2003; Frith 2004; Klin 2000; Trillingsgaard 1999).

One psychiatrist recalls a discussion with a 15-year-old boy with AS about the reasons for people marrying. He was so impressed with the boy's analysis that he hastily began scribbling it down, thinking he might email it to several friends later on. However, at the end of the session the counterbalance in the boy's poor nonverbal communication, lack of eye contact and 'abruptness' in leaving the room underlined the profound bifurcation between his intellect and lived experience.

The adolescent with AS

Typical adolescent development is much different from childhood development. As a child enters adolescence, the features that define childhood play give way to more sophisticated communication about areas of joint interest. Gradually this develops into communication about common values, rather than common interests. In a few short years, an individual has moved from being a child interested in a specific toy to an adolescent experimenting with politics, religion and relationships. The transition is rapid and challenging, even for the most capable.

Adolescence is a time of multiple rapid transitions and poses a range of different challenges for everyone. Developmental stages dictate that, along with handling daily stresses, the typical adolescent must:

- cope with profound personal physiological changes

- develop a sexual identity and orientation

- build up a social identity

- manage peer relationships largely unmonitored by parents

- accept greater cognitive demands at school

- develop employment and career goals

- begin laying the foundations for an independent life separate from his or her parents.

A therapist must factor all of these developmental events into the structure of an intervention. The intervention must not only reference where the group is 'at' developmentally, but also where their peers are 'at'.

What is the impact of AS on everyday adolescent life? The transition through adolescence is frequently emotionally and psychologically distressing. Bullying, social exclusion and ridicule are very common experiences for a child with AS. The extent to which adolescents with AS will pretend to fit in though they are deeply unhappy inside has been documented by several sources (Carrington and Graham 2001; Church, Alisanski and Amanuallah 2000).

Additional difficulties revolve around immature, absent or mainly negative peer relations resulting in isolation, victimisation and lack of peer support. Self-organisational difficulties, low self-esteem, depression and anxiety are further compounding problems for adolescents with AS. These experiences influence the intervention dynamics. For example, discussion of topics that might give offence or stimulate anxious thoughts must be handled reassuringly. It is important to remember that adolescence for those with AS is not an impossible obstacle. Many successfully go to college and find employment.

Identifying AS: assessment before group therapy is crucial

Those with AS do not form a strongly homogenous group, which is another of its puzzling features. Some may have poor eye contact in conversation, while others may have excellent eye contact. Some may have a distinct monotone voice, while others have close to typical prosody. Meeting the diagnostic criteria is often all they have in common. This can be confusing at times for inexperienced professionals who occasionally will not be able to identify that a patient has Asperger syndrome even after a number of conversations.

> Tim was 14 years old. He had normal intonation and prosody in his speech, good eye contact and was polite and willing to respond to questions. In a group setting, he did not hang back from the others, but joined them in conversation at break time. The only marked peculiarity of his conversation occurred when asked to converse with other group members. He found the initiation of conversation difficult. When asked to be a respondent in a conversation, he invariably answered his interlocutor with lists of statements. He appeared to have little comprehension of either the importance of coherence in conversation, or the value in paying attention to his audience's reactions. Despite these demonstrated peculiarities, it would have been difficult to conclude that Tim had Asperger syndrome without access to assessments and a clinical history.

Once AS is suspected then a detailed clinical history is required to confirm the diagnosis in all cases. Screening for associated conditions should take place. A therapist should always study the clinical history of group participants before assembling an intervention. Combining clinically mismatched populations may lead to lack of focus and uneven progress. Reinforcing this caveat, Gillberg (2002) reports that a group functions best when matched for intelligence levels and general functioning, otherwise it may collapse.

Determining the functional, expressive and receptive language abilities of individual participants prior to group selection informs the delivery and interactions. Therapists with a speech and language background will presumably make more of this information than those whose training is more general. Unfortunately, accurate measures of more generalised linguistic communication deficits – the pragmatic communication deficits – are not easy to obtain. A number of studies have commented on the implications of the lack of standardised social communication assessment instruments for the adolescent group (Adams 2002; Adams et al. 2002; Koning and Magill-Evans 2001; Landa 2000; Rinaldi 2001). Partly because of this gap, a participant with a suspected diagnosis of Asperger syndrome may be admitted to an intervention, but without a full psychological assessment.

Jack joined a social competence intervention group because of a suspected diagnosis of Asperger syndrome. Subsequent psychological testing indicated that he was functioning in the mild learning disability range, especially in expressive and functional language comprehension and performance. However, he was now de facto in the intervention group. He was a quiet 15-year-old boy and always attempted to verbalise answers to questions. On average, however, each interaction with Jack could take between six and ten times longer than with other group members. In practice, this meant that six members of the group could complete separate interactions with the therapist in the time Jack could complete one. The only method that could assist both the group and Jack was to devise fewer questions for him, with a short answer focus. Typically, he would be asked either yes/no questions or else 'fill in the blank' questions.

The situation described with Jack should never arise, but limited assessment resources and parental pressure for assistance may sometimes cause the premature placement of an individual in an intervention. The participant may derive very little benefit from the direct verbal and written content of an intervention. Role-play opportunities are also limited. If the participant is enjoying himself with his peers in the group, then that is something not to be set aside lightly. It is a measure of progress. The therapist has to balance the amount of time that each participant requires against the requirements of other group members. Opportunities for developing social contacts within the group should not be underestimated, As long as a participant is not disruptive there is an arguable therapeutic case for retaining him or her in the group.

Social skills, social cognition and social competence

One can flounder under a deluge of technical terminology when discussing social skills training and autistic spectrum disorders in tandem. Frequently, the technical terminology is actually the clearest expression of the main substance behind a concept, method or principle. It helps categorise components and features for examination. This also helps us work out whether we are comparing like with like, rather than simply putting an ad hoc analysis together. The terminology helps to pin down the significant features of communication and interaction that need to be made explicit for those with AS.

Any useful intervention makes explicit what is implicit in everyday interaction. Various philosophical theories about communication, language and mind have analysed implicit characteristics of everyday life over many decades. The business of philosophy is about stating the obvious and examining our assumptions around what it is to be 'obvious'. Although the media constantly confuses woolly mysticism with academic philosophy, a therapist should not. Under examination, many of the key features of autistic spectrum disorders have useful philosophical resonances – they can have a practical impact on interventions. An effective intervention for AS adolescents is one that helps them practically to apply the materials. Later, in Chapter 3, we discuss effective communication. We trace a route that follows practical steps from the philosophy of language into speech and language studies and on into psychiatry. Applying philosophical insights will not seem at all puzzling then.

Childhood autism interventions

The phrase social skills training (SST) is commonly used to describe interventions that are (a) geared to correct or compensate for the social deficits of a person; (b) intended to enhance a person's existing social skills and provide new ones. The skills are 'new' in the sense of being ones that the subject would not have employed before. A persistent concern in SST, especially with autistic children, is the extent to which the skills learned generalise to the outside world, if at all (Barry, et al. 2003; Hadwin et al. 1997; Ozonoff and Miller 1995; Rogers 2000). Several autobiographies by people with AS record difficulties in attempting to (or forgetting to) generalise social skills in adolescence (Gerland 1997; Grandin and Scariano 1986; Holliday Willey 1999; Jackson 2002; Shore 2003). Adolescent interventions must also address the generalisation problem that is common in child-focused interventions. The goal of any socialisation intervention is to effect changes in social behaviour that generalise beyond the setting of the group. This objective must be to the forefront of the therapist's mind in delivering and evaluating the group intervention.

The efficacy of an intervention should be relatively easy to identify and measure in theory – 'There he is. He is using what he has learnt, and he never did that before.' A review of SSTs for children with behavioural and emotional problems found striking inconsistencies in the effectiveness of SSTs for a variety of reasons (Spence 2003). Improvements where they occur may be transient, affect only a limited number of behaviours, or fail to generalise. For example, one intervention dealing with victims of bullying, a familiar theme in AS, revealed that improvements in self-esteem were disappointingly not matched by improvements in other areas of social functioning (Fox and Boulton 2003). Evaluations of SSTs for children do not automatically cover adolescent interventions for developmental reasons touched on above. One could argue that evaluations of SSTs for non-autistic children may have scant relevance for autistic spectrum centred interventions. The question is how should these results influence thinking on SSTs for adolescents with AS? There is no easy answer to this question. As an attempt at a broad response, a brief account of the intervention situation in childhood autism is worth recounting.

Relevant interventions involve social skills training pitched at developmentally appropriate standards. Efforts to meet the educational and social needs of autistic children are based on the principle that early intervention is best, (National Research Council 2001). For example, an intervention for an eight-year-old is much different from that for a three-year-old. The same report by the US National Research Council reviewed ten educational interventions. It noted a wide range of differing and often conflicting evaluation measures used to measure the outcomes of interventions (in other words, their value to the participants). It was difficult to be certain that like was being compared with like when comparing the various interventions.

The variation between interventions underlines just how difficult it is to reach agreement on even a framework for social skills training. No one-size-fits-all approach was identified or recommended in the report. This is not a criticism of the interventions but an acknowledgement of the complexity of the task of teaching the 'obvious' to these children.

When we look for developmentally appropriate interventions for the AS adolescent, the range of options is actually worse in comparison with childhood autism. There are surprisingly few well-developed evaluations of interventions for AS adolescents. Given the variety of social skills interventions being marketed, how do we explain this anomaly?

AS in adolescence: intervention caveats and core themes

Clinical experience and research indicate that treatment for the AS adolescent group as a whole has lagged behind those with more pronounced global learning impairments. One explanation offered is that the apparent near 'normality' of the AS adolescent group places added pressure on them to 'fit in' and incomprehension among others when they do not (Attwood 1998; Howlin 1998). As a result, because of their good verbal ability, their needs are perceived as more marginal.

For instance, in one school known to the authors a senior teacher was quite insistent that an adolescent with AS was 'shirking' and should 'just get on with it'. When dealing with other problematic adolescents, this teacher was very understanding but he could not grasp AS. This reaction is not uncommon. The quandary for the person with AS is that his or her near normality may militate against them getting the necessary assistance and support in the school environment. A therapist should obtain a school history for each participant. Otherwise, the intervention may begin with assumptions about school support (reasonable assumptions, by the way) that are simply misleading.

Bauminger notes research suggesting that the problems children with high-functioning autism experience with peers (social initiation and socioemotional understanding) may be misunderstood as evidence of social insensitivity and disinterest (Bauminger 2002). Adolescents with AS may be perceived as intentionally hostile, indifferent or dismissive. Understandable as this is from within the typical peer system of social values, the attribution of intentionality to those with AS should always be considered as the last explanatory option, not the first. This is a practical rule of thumb for every therapist.

The use of the phrase social skills training (SST) is so entrenched in practice that invariably all socialisation interventions are assumed to be skills focused. A number of qualms can be raised against describing social competence building interventions as social skills interventions. In the first place, the concept of a social skill is not well defined. If we describe someone as a skilled mathematician or a skilled block layer, we can generally point to measurable aspects of their behaviour that reveal their excellence. For example, we refer to people being skilled negotiators on the evidence that they are knowledgeable about the effective use of persuasive strategies. However, who could list all the presumed skills they use?

Second, one cannot learn a language by learning lists of sentences, any more than one can learn enough 'social skills' by learning a list of micro-skills. Rote learning of skill steps has a role in child centred interventions, but a lesser one in adolescent-centred interventions. In the latter group, differentiation between skills and the force with which they are expressed in given circumstances determines effective interactions.

Third, social skills are *behaviours* that are publicly observable and directed towards someone else, e.g. greeting, listening, acknowledging, thanking, and so forth (it would be next to impossible to annotate every social skill). A behavioural component with a purpose is necessary in an SST intervention to develop practical communication and interaction strategies.

Finally, social learning involves more than understanding the bare set of conditions for deploying a skill. It also involves *judging* how to deploy the skill successfully. Differentiation between various social and emotional factors in interpersonal situations is essential. Knowing how to ask for help is one thing. Knowing how to ask for help tactfully is quite something else. In practice this means that any intervention for adolescents with AS must have both behavioural and cognitive components, that is, a component that deals with how people think and make judgements about communication and interaction.

In summary, having social skills is one thing, but judging when and how best to deploy them is entirely different. Any intervention should have a cognitive-behavioural approach to ground both the modelling and assessment of communication and interaction events. Therefore, for these reasons, the use of social skills training is a misnomer. Therapists may continue to use the phrase for convenience and because it has such wide currency, but an effective intervention must go beyond conventional social skills only approaches.

A more apposite phrase is *social competence*. It embraces the idea of social performance (the behaviours) and judgement about the delivery and objectives of the performance (the social cognitive judgement and emotion processing). It also blends the dual aims of generating the essentials for (a) behaviours that will lead to successful social outcomes; and (b) abilities to combine cognitive, emotional and behavioural skills flexibly depending on social context and demands.

Interventions must avoid the production of socially competent hermits. If that is the outcome of an intervention then it cannot be judged successful. Interventions must orient towards interpersonal interactions, always shifting the focus between cognitive comprehension and physical modelling of the topics – *Think then Do!* The emphasis on interactivity is fundamental. Without modelling interaction themes (or where modelling opportunities are limited), there is a risk that participants will merely internalise social skills as an intellectual skill. In that case, the intervention is an empty exercise.

One of the authors recalls an occasion when an adolescent with AS dismissed the need for practice on the grounds that he had read the book and could 'write essays on it'.

Social competence does not imply social perfection; no more than having a competence with language marks everyone as a skilled negotiator or brilliant wit. What defines a person's social competence is not his own evaluation of his social interaction skills. The evaluations and responses of others in different social contexts are critical. Adolescents with AS should be taught that social competence is defined by the extent to which their social interactions and outcomes with other people are mutually satisfactory and positive. We rely on reciprocation (in initiation and response) to determine the quality of interpersonal communication. This is a core theme for any AS-focused intervention and needs constant elaboration and reinforcement by a therapist – a point that cannot be overstated.

Therapists have to set reasonable standards based on group assessment and progress. Otherwise, they may set unreasonable standards for the group. Having a large bundle of materials for an intervention should not dictate the speed of the intervention. Therapists, especially those from a teaching background, find this troubling. They are accustomed to equating competence with getting the materials across to their group. This approach is too rigid with AS adolescents (we return to defining just what is reasonable in Chapter 6). Figure 1.1 presents the core themes and their relationships in an intervention concentrated on enhancing social interaction abilities.

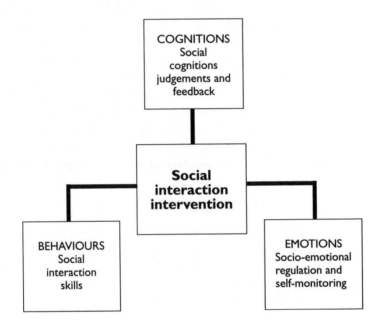

Figure 1.1 Core themes and relationships in an intervention to enhance social interaction abilities

Susan Spence (2003) argues that the promise that SST held out 30 years ago has been tempered by the gradual realisation that its benefits are most noticeable as a component integrated into sophisticated cognitive-behavioural interventions. Spence's review does not address AS explicitly but notes general observations about SST. She lists ten components that inform social competence. Adolescents with AS have difficulties in all the areas listed:

1.   Interpersonal problem-solving skills.

2.   Accurate processing of social information.

3. Social perception and perspective taking.

4. Cognitive distortion and maladaptive thinking styles.

5. Social knowledge.

6. Environmental contingencies for social responding.

7. Social opportunities for modelling and teaching of pro-social skills by others.

8. Emotion regulation (e.g. anxiety and anger management).

9. Self-regulation and self-monitoring.

10. Ability to perform social skills.

None of these components could be reduced to simple skills. Social skills are rarely atomic acts. They result from combining lower order verbal and nonverbal skills. It is precisely here that AS adolescents' generalisation abilities break down. For instance, an AS adolescent may learn the micro-skills behind, say, asking for help – a macro-level social skill – but fail to combine the micro-skills consistently. At a nonverbal level, these include eye contact, tone of voice, posture, expression and appropriate proximity. Verbally, tone of voice, synchronisation of delivery and volume may be inappropriate and out of step with the style of language. The macro-level social skill may not be realised because the purpose of the macro-skill is unclear.

The distinction between macro- and micro-skills is analogous to that between a goal and the plan required to realise it. Other macro-skills include greeting someone, responding to a criticism, initiating a conversation, and so forth. Traditionally, macro-level skills have been associated with communication themes, while micro-level skills are seen as lower order behavioural components that operationalise the macro-skill. Transference, or carryover, of 'skills' is problematic.

Michael had been diagnosed with AS at the age of ten. His progress through secondary school was steady. He had a supportive secondary school environment, including a special 'disability' room with resource teacher. Among his classmates, he was accepted but had no friendships with them. He tended to 'make friends' among the new yearly intake who were generally three to four years younger. This caused problems on occasions as the younger ones would make fun of him by imitating his gestures or hiding his bag. After a series of such episodes, he was advised by the resource teacher not to speak to the younger students. Michael duly followed these instructions. Instead, he would wait outside school for the others and hand them letters he had written explaining his current thinking. Unfortunately, the younger students found this form of communication unnerving. Eventually, following a complaint, Michael was told not to contact the others at any time or using any means.

Michael's case illustrates a major challenge facing any intervention – concrete literal reasoning. Michael was told not to initiate contact by speech but no one mentioned that written communication was also out of bounds.

Concrete thinking about social problems may occasionally appear subversive, but literal thinking is a hallmark of AS and any reliance by a therapist on typical implicit social conventions (inferences) to guide social behaviour will probably fail. Drilling the adolescent to demonstrate a social skill in one setting does not guarantee that conventional associated skills will be learnt at all. This is the reason why developing AS adolescents' social cognitions is so important to aid their judgements in solving social problems. It is also another reason why the instructional skills of inspirational therapists are hard to capture and relay efficiently to others.

Problem factors

Two additional factors that influence the uptake of 'standard' social skill training as applied to AS are:

- the need for concrete explanations for adopting particular cognitions and skills

- the depressive or unmotivated outlook of many adolescents with AS.

Regarding the first factor, scientific justifications for social contact, such as group and teamwork, may be useful, if at times slightly controversial. For example, one could use an evolutionary argument in favour of participative teamwork because it guarantees species survival. Failure to provide justifications for the choices of theme, topic or method may undermine the intervention. Occasionally justifications may not be 'good enough' for the AS group. Rather than becoming defensive, a therapist may need to return with a more sound justification. Appealing to authority is not a useful justification strategy, especially if the goal is to persuade the participants of the wisdom of one's arguments. It is unclear whether justifications based solely in moral norms are convincing.

Asserting that it is *'nice to be with people'* or it is *'good to help other people'* may be entirely inadequate to an AS adolescent who rejects associations between facts and values. A more useful approach is to dwell on the benefit to the participant of the attitude/behaviour. For example: *'If you help someone else, they will probably like you better and are more likely to help you in the future.'* You may also feel good inside by showing that you can help another person.

The second factor is more complex and we just touch on it for the moment. The question is not whether depressed or unmotivated AS adolescents should participate in interventions, but whether they will 'pull down' group dynamics. Such adolescents may have a history of adverse social reactions. Social contexts have become sources of immense anxiety. Their willingness, even minimally, to initiate social interactions may be absent. A change in social perception and thinking must be effected. The phrase 'cognitive restructuring' is often used to refer to a process by which a participant learns to think about situations differently. It implies learning to interpret the social world differently and one's reactions to it. This relies very much on identifying implicit features of a situation that had gone unnoticed before and 'bringing them up' for evaluation. For instance, in trying to understand someone's behaviour, we have to ask ourselves why the behaviour is displayed, rather than simply making a judgement about it. In order to change one's behaviour, the thinking behind the behaviour (if there is any) must also change. Bringing about a shift in perspective is crucial in dealing with AS misperceptions of the social world.

Interpersonal problem solving is underdeveloped in AS (failure to learn from past social experiences and reactions is common). Ineffective social responses continue unmodified in the absence of appropriate feedback and assessment. Without intervention, this amounts to doing the same thing repeatedly. It happens that AS adolescents may find themselves mixing with inappropriate company but not know how to avoid continuously being in the 'wrong' company. There are a number of explanations, but deviant peer groups may attract the marginalised peer. A deviant peer group that is uninterested in typical social conventions can be appealing.

A proper appreciation of the AS adolescent's inability to extract accurate social knowledge about others and their interpersonal relationships is essential to managing any intervention. Developing alternative social strategies with accompanying predictions and consequence evaluation are exceptionally inhibited without this knowledge. Reasoning about social interaction strategies should be developed and practised in any intervention: *Doing must be supported by Thinking.*

Social competence intervention methods

Categorisations of the components of SSTs (whether in broad or thin forms) have been developed in a number of works and it is important that a therapist grasp them as useful tools for structuring the intervention. A constant focus on peer–peer interactions both within and outside the group must be maintained at all times. We have drawn on a number of sources including our own practices in presenting the components which are important in an intervention (Attwood 2000; Baron-Cohen 2004; Bauminger 2002; Bock 2001; Cook 2002; Frith 2004; Greenway 2000; Hanko 1999; Harpur *et al.* 2003; Klin and Volkmar 2000; Rogers 2000; Sirota 2004; Spence 2003; Trillingsgaard 1999; Vaughn and Lancelotta 1990; Whitehill, Hersen and Bellack 1980).

Behaviour-focused methods

In what follows, we talk about learning behaviours, but you can equally interpret references to behaviours as roughly equivalent to talk of social skills. Giving directions, promoting discussions and modelling different skills form the core methods for introducing social interactions. Modelling of skills is undertaken by the therapist and usually an assistant. Modelling ineffective behaviours should be counterbalanced with modelling effective behaviours. The AS group explores what is ineffective about a particular behaviour and then moves towards modelling effective behaviours. This method aids a group to understand and practise eye contact, for example.

Initiating behaviours should be addressed first – getting the attention of others. Logically, the continuance of an interaction is reliant on first making contact with another person. A clear explanation for the behaviours should be offered to the group. A therapist should not presume that members of the group have grasped sequencing of actions. Responding behaviours are equally important and teaching initiation–response paired behaviour is a precursor to introducing reciprocation – the process of responding to a social action with an appropriate corresponding one. The group will need these core behaviours referenced at every session.

The development of a participant's social skills is rooted in him or her rehearsing the skills in the group setting. Typically, this involves role play. The participant plays the role of either an initiator or a responder. Roles that are more complex are present in everyday interactions but a basic grounding in initiation–response skills is essential for communication and social integration. Practice in the group elicits feedback from the therapist, the group and the participant. Feedback should always be constructive and encouraging. Group discussions and feedback help reinforce positive social cognitions and behaviours. In turn, these aid the development of alternative communication strategies and problem solving skills. Social behaviour is always directed behaviour. It has a purpose, and the AS adolescent must explicitly be helped to derive that purpose in a social setting for the behaviour to apply.

Social blindness and peer expectations

Interpreting social cues and nuances is an area of extreme weakness in AS adolescents. They are 'blind' to them. When should I greet someone? How do I greet them? Am I greeting the right sort of person? These are puzzling questions for someone with AS.

Descriptions and justifications of social activities are necessary for AS adolescents. Frequently, they do not apprehend the social context supporting communication. Emphasising, with clear examples, that certain contexts have minimum sets of rules is necessary. For example, in school it is accepted that students do not interrupt the teacher or interfere with other students. In explaining these rules to AS adolescents, who may not 'see' them, one might be called upon to justify them rationally.

A therapist should distinguish between existing practices (which fall short of a desired high standard) and expected practices. These efforts should be supported by modelling and rehearsal. However, the focus here is largely cognitive in that the group is asked to analyse and 'think through' social encounters as the precursor to formulating strategies and reactions. Methods should focus on cue identification, elaboration of peer expectations and self/other emotions in context. Drawing the participants into their own group discussions and explorations of these issues facilitates conversation and inter alia exposure and practice around the topics of importance.

Video modelling (with appropriate scripts) has proved a useful tool in exploring ineffective and effective social interactions in a range of situations (Dowrick 1986). Video character cognitions and emotions can be explored and discussed to create improved solution-focused role play in the group. One of the major deficits in AS is an uneven grasp (if at all) of the expectations of peers. Getting across to people with AS that other people in the world are as important as they are can be very thorny. It is important to emphasise repeatedly that peers have expectations about interactions – about how interactions should begin, proceed and end. A therapist will spend much time reiterating this point. It is important to help the group discuss how the common ground between people helps communication. People with AS tend not to 'see' the common ground. They need help in formulating strategies to derive what is common between them and whoever they are interacting with. Later on in the book we examine a range of strategies that therapists can use here.

Identification of contingencies and emotions

The AS reaction to change (stress) is rooted in a reluctance to have the predictability of one set of circumstances replaced by the unpredictability of another.

Everyday life is dynamic and changes in time, place and company are unavoidable. Most typical people manage the dynamics of everyday life with relative ease. Their capacity to accommodate changes in routine is not overtaxed. If the unexpected occurs (unless it is extreme) people adjust and develop alternative plans. This capacity to deal with the unexpected through the generation of alternative plans is intrinsic to the process of *contingency management* – our definition is different from the definition used in behavioural therapies. Allowing for, and responding to, contingencies are dispositions that people with AS find challenging to develop and practise. Often they are overwhelmed.

Discussion of contingencies, as unexpected events or interruptions to a routine or plan, is best explored through some form of counterfactual reasoning based on 'what-if' analysis. In our case, we make use of video scenario discussions extensively. After a video scenario is played to the group, the options open to characters (verbal, nonverbal and emotional) are discussed. They are then further analysed by asking the group to tease out the implications for characters if one of them was other than portrayed, for example, 'What if he said X, then how would…?'

It is important to steer participants away from 'dead-end' reasoning that interferes with learning new cognitive styles. In the beginning, participants may answer with more 'I don't knows' than anything else. This can be frustrating but gentle prompting to produce at least one definite outcome option should be pursued. Working in parallel with the methods cited above, the concentration is on comprehending and then modelling the contingency management strategies of others (these can be video characters).

The possibility of change is gradually opened up. This can be continued through into role play that rehearses coping with change, disappointment and outcome failures. Feedback should be sensitively phrased since contingency management is immensely challenging for all those with AS. The role played by the emotions in helping to execute a successful interaction is a key quality. A 'bad' emotional reaction tends to close down peer interactions. Aligning contingency management with emotion regulation has benefits. It connects communicative purpose and outcomes with emotion states. It also leads into exploring emotions in others and the point in responding appropriately – empathy. Extensive modelling and role play are required since self and other emotion recognition is decidedly impaired in AS (Hill, Berthoz and Frith 2004).

Self-monitoring and self-regulation methods
Self-instructional methods are helpful in teaching relaxation exercises for anger and anxiety management. In turn, these support personal and social problem

solving. The idea behind these methods is to teach participants to think through solutions 'out loud' and then over time internalise this thinking (Camp and Bash 1981). The therapy is used commonly to train individuals to manage anger or a conduct disorder. Usually the therapist will model a solution to a problem by talking the participants through the solution. This process is then continued by the participants and finally, after much practice, they continue with internal dialogues. The extent to which traditional think aloud therapy can be used effectively in the group is related to its size. It may be impractical in a large group.

In the case of AS think aloud strategies can help participants learn to think through rules for social interaction before committing. This will amount to recalling the steps required for the situation. Again this method, like so many other stepwise methods, must be knitted in with unfolding higher social cognitive processing. This is essential for developing social competence and generalisation strategies. The methods can also be used to encourage participants to speak out a solution or speak their mind constructively in the initial sessions while participants are coming to terms with each other's company and proximity.

We have used a rule for the initial sessions emphasising that in verbal interactions *quantity is better than quality*. This aims to encourage self-expression and self-monitoring during a crucial phase in building a 'safe place' for the group. One participant was troubled by the 'quantity' component since it appeared to inveigh against what he had learnt elsewhere. He was right of course, but the aim of the rule is to encourage contributions in the session as a foundation for building relations with other participants.

Once participants have learnt to relax with one another, the 'quantity is better than quality' rule is given up in place of a *be relevant* rule. Instruction in self-regulation (emotion and stress regulation) is important when dealing with AS adolescents. Any form of social skills training needs to be grounded in participant relaxation. Without relaxed participants, the sessions will be at the least ineffective and at the worst stress heightening. Visualisation exercises are helpful, but should be thoroughly explained to the group. One that we have found particularly effective is given in Appendix 1.

Problem solving: interpersonal and social

Teaching interpersonal problem-solving skills involves helping participants to identify problem social situations, appropriate strategies and alternatives, and finally a means for assessing the efficacy of any interaction. Rational problem-solving strategies must always be put forward in a group intervention for AS.

Self-instruction is usually a component of any training. With AS adolescents it is important to present more rather than less problematic scenarios for resolution. This requirement arises from the generalisation impairments whereby the solution for one context may not generalise to another, despite similarities. The need to be explicit in giving directions, presenting strategies and insisting on role play cannot be understated. For instance, it is common for adolescents with AS to give perfectly adequate verbal solutions but be unable to put these into practice – develop the behavioural expressions. Social problem solving has to be grounded in practice. Second, suggesting that participants learn by observing other peers may not be helpful unless they are advanced in their understanding of nonverbal communication and appropriate boundaries – if they are that advanced why are they in the intervention?

The 'boundary problem' is one that parents report as giving many difficulties, especially if the adolescent is attracted to deviant peer groups. In those situations, explaining why he or she needs to avoid the deviant group is challenging and fractious for parents. Taking these issues into a group setting is equally knotty. Therapists should be cautious when responding to parental agendas within the intervention group. Preferably, the issues should emerge during the course of discussions. For example, discussions could be centred on friendship and responsibility and the problem solving skills required to maintain both.

Problem solving in general

Problem solving, whether at the level of self-regulation or interpersonal, should emphasise refining a problem situation into steps. Break each problem into smaller bits. The refinement process is a precursor to a strategy that leads to a solution. In practise, this means recognising the problem for what it is and then generating a *planned* response – not an impulsive response.

Assessing the efficacy of a response is complicated for AS adolescents due to impaired 'reading' of other people. Often a bare minimum response may be considered perfectly adequate to an autistic person with an attendant 'pared down psyche'. It can be difficult to persuade AS adolescents to move beyond the bare response. One is trying to persuade them that a bare response is less effective in interactions. Persuading the AS adolescent to offer more than the bare response requires persuading him or her that there is greater benefit in doing so. Modelling, video analysis and role play are extremely advantageous.

Expanding the response repertoire will require that participants explore peer expectations in detail. Behaviour is again to be guided by social cognitive processing. The dilemma faced by a therapist is on the one hand encouraging adequate interaction content, while on the other discouraging prolixity and irrelevance. We look at these issues in more detail in Chapter 3.

> Ben had been diagnosed with AS at the age of ten. He had attended a number of SST interventions. He progressed through secondary school without making friends. His classmates accepted that he was 'different'. Fortunately, the school he attended had a robust anti-bullying policy. Reports from his parents and teachers revealed that peers found conversing with Ben impossible. Ben tended to interject in every conversation by plucking a detail and then relating it exclusively to something in his personal experience. Peers judged that Ben was uninterested in their experiences. His experiences were more important than theirs were. Consequently, peers avoided his company.

How could Ben be helped? In the first place, Ben needed coaching in active listening. Time should be set aside in each session to rehearse the rules and goals of active listening (we go through these again in the chapters on the intervention template). Many AS adolescents have problems paying appropriate attention to sufficient details in an interaction. This difficulty is intrinsic to AS. Second, speaking out is not equivalent to communication. The latter requires getting and holding the attention of an audience. Typical peers manifest this through the *intentionality* behind their communications. Most people understand this implicitly: people with AS need to be taught it. Third, Ben needed help to explore the expectations of typical peers that are relevant to successful interactions. People with AS often view communication purely as information exchange, and in certain contexts that is appropriate. However, typical peer-to-peer social interaction is also about sharing and exploring each other's social identities – *get to know one another.* Finally, the AS worldview is largely egocentric in which the limits of experience tend to be perceived as the limits of the AS person's experience. Other people mistakenly perceive this attitude as dismissive, rude and selfish. Helping Ben to see the world differently entails educating him to understand these problems. This entails educating him in social experimentation strategies that will help him recognise and process feedback usefully. Ultimately, a different set of cognitive principles and behavioural skills for addressing social interactions are required. While laboratory acquisition of many of these features is viable, extending these to the external world is an entirely different matter. Despite extensive coaching, Ben will continue to have difficulties managing competing/inhibiting/inappropriate responses. The aim is to lessen the difficulties and their impact on him and other peers. Note that therapists running socialisation interventions have huge responsibilities.

None of these tasks is remotely trivial. One cannot expect to end the AS perspective on the world and produce a 'typical' person. However, one can reasonably hope to mend aspects of the AS perspective in many cases.

Efficacy of social skills training interventions

This is perhaps the biggest issue concerning any SST related intervention. While a number of studies are available for young autistic children, there are few available for AS adolescents. 'How effective is intervention X?' When faced with this question, therapists are faced with answering a question that is largely meaningless in the absence of studies of standardised content and delivery. Spence (2003) in her review cites a number of studies that question the efficacy of SSTs in general – mainly due to inconsistencies among participant characteristics, types of intervention, measures used, and the assessment of short-term and long-term generalisations. The lack of consistent high quality data on interventions compels the therapist to fall back on best practice models and the preferences of more experienced colleagues.

Multimodal strengths and weaknesses

Social skills and social problem solving interventions are increasingly using multimodal delivery paths to enhance their efficacy. Parents, teachers and peers are recruited as social agents that facilitate the 'roll out' of the intervention with adolescents. The delivery modes involve more than therapist–group interaction. A number of multimodal interventions have been tried with young autistic children as reported by the National Research Council. Much less is known about the impact of similar interventions for AS adolescents (Bauminger being a notable exception). For a whole range of reasons outside the therapist's control, the operation of a multimodal intervention can oscillate wildly. A therapist must decide what minimum level of multimodality is achievable consistently and plan accordingly.

The use of school peers in supportive roles has the potential benefit of drawing the AS adolescent into interaction with peers. The 'buddy system' and 'circle of friends' have been tried in a number of individual education plans (IEPs) whereby the AS adolescent has a series of 'social chaperones' in the school environment. A number of practitioners very strongly favour this approach. In the absence of long-term studies of groups, the evidence in favour is largely based on individual reports and clinical judgement (Moyes 2001; Myles and Adreon 2001; Ozonoff, Dawson and McPartland 2002). Reservations about this approach include that peers will not be equipped to meet the demands of the AS adolescent consistently, and the provision of regular support for befrienders will be overlooked. It is usual for school-based interventions to include teacher-training components. Teachers, rather than specialist therapists, will more than likely be those delivering a school-based intervention. Their monitoring of the AS adolescent in a peer environment is an advantage when assembling observations and reports. In addition, teachers are usually the first contact for school incidents involving peers and AS adolescents. Despite these advantages, the instructional methods of conventional teaching do not readily lend themselves to social skills training and social problem solving.

The blending of parents into interventions requires careful consideration of their role. The tasks and their impact are different from those assigned to the adolescents. It is necessary not only to provide information (feedback) to parents but also give them structured directions to learn and practise with their children.

Parents can play a significant role in interventions aimed at children with conduct disorder or who are socially excluded (Frankel, Cantwell and Myatt 1996; Frankel et al. 1997; Kazadin 1997). The involvement of parents, in the case of AS, must be weighed against:

- the capacity of parents to meet intervention objectives given their everyday family and work responsibilities

- the presence of autistic traits in the parents themselves.

The first is a general rule applying to all socialisation interventions, but the second case is particular to autistic spectrum interventions. A range of studies show that the parents of autistic spectrum children often exhibit autistic traits themselves (Landa, Folstein and Isaacs 1991; Landa et al. 1992; O'Hanrahan and Fitzgerald 1999; Piven, Chase et al. 1991). Expectations of parents should be tempered and one should not assume these parents can contribute the input that typical parents might.

Overview of the book

Adolescence is a very troubling time for those with AS. Even if social skills interventions have been available at elementary and primary school level, the radical nature of adolescent transformations, especially in communication, provides sufficient grounds for an adolescent-focused intervention. The approach outlined here is based on identifying preferred outcomes and then working towards them using triads of Theme–Topic–Method while working with the expectations of group.

The methodology of the intervention is also multimodal in that parental participation is intrinsic to it and peer participation is desirable. It is compatible with the materials produced in many social skills interventions that are currently circulating. The aim of this book is to help the therapist (or parent) make the right choice of materials be they from one or twenty interventions, and only then folding the materials into a targeted intervention for his or her own group of AS adolescents. Despite the plethora of interventions, there are sound reasons for following this approach. These include the influence of cultural factors, the uneven presentation of AS and the often mixed background that therapists have themselves. This is an attempt to set down criteria for social competence interventions based on a collection of methodological and best practice principles discussed in the text.

The aim of this chapter was to give therapists a footing in the debate about interventions for AS adolescents. It is a complex area. In addition, we flagged our own focus on educating intervention participants in recognising peer expectations and the behaviours necessary for effective social interaction. We reiterate that the primary objective of any intervention for AS adolescents is to push theory into peer interactions for the benefit of the AS adolescent. All social skill related interventions must support peer interactions.

We amplify these points systematically in the remaining chapters, beginning with an outline of current thinking about AS and its implications for social interaction interventions. This is followed by a brief chapter on communication and language issues in AS. We make extensive use of case studies here to illustrate our arguments. Next, we describe our own intervention template for a social interaction intervention. We flag the importance of psycho-social assessment of participants prior to joining an intervention. Since video modelling and the use of ineffective/effective scripts play a large role in our own intervention, we devoted a chapter to describing the components. Good housekeeping dictated that we outline session formats, problems and solutions that therapists may find helpful. The penultimate chapter discusses session plans and how they are delivered. Finally, we conclude with a chapter on evaluation and the challenges involved.

2 Current Thinking on Asperger Syndrome

This chapter presents an overview of aspects of current research and thinking on Asperger syndrome. We present the theories and ideas to help the reader reference several core principles in the social interaction therapy intervention. Although it is widely accepted in the research community that autistic spectrum disorders are both neurodevelopmental in origin and strongly linked to genetic inheritance the current neuroscientific and psychological understanding of AS is incomplete. The rich descriptions of symptoms and their associations give valuable partial insights into what may underlie AS but they do not provide a cause-and-effect explanation for it. Perhaps, from a therapeutic perspective, one of the most important facts to bear in mind about AS is that some very intellectually able people (as measured by traditional IQ tests) may demonstrate very poor socio-emotional understanding and a very limited repertoire of socially adaptive behaviour. To confuse matters further, social deficits are not evenly distributed in AS. What exactly does this mean? Consider a simple analogy for the moment. Imagine that social interaction capacities of adolescents could be laid along a developmental timeline. We might get something like Figure 2.1.

The typical peer has more of whatever makes him or her socially adaptive. The AS adolescent peer has 'less' of the necessary capacities. If the pictures overleaf were accurate, social deficits would be fixed by topping up with the missing capacities. However, research and clinical practice indicate that this linear one-dimensional model does not capture the unevenness of social disabilities in AS (Gillberg 2002; Klin *et al.* 2000). A more plausible account is that the capacities and disabilities vary along a range of dimensions, and vary between persons with AS. For instance, comprehending tone of voice may pose problems for some with AS but not others. The same applies to facial expression recognition, eye contact, vocal expression, fondness for sport, comprehension of narratives, and so forth. Hence, it is not just the variation in abilities but also the variation in their distribution that poses numerous scientific and therapeutic challenges.

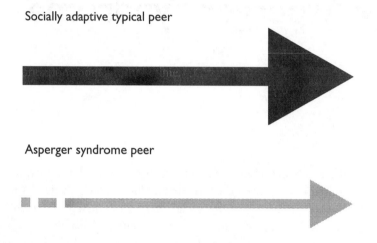

Figure 2.1 Social interaction capacities of adolescents on developmental timeline

Historically, explanations for autism have drawn on diverse sources. The earliest explanation and now most discredited, blamed the condition on a mother's inability to form appropriate attachment relations with her child. The 'refrigerator mother' and 'empty fortress' theories attributed the withholding of motherly love as the primary factor in accounting for autism (Bettleheim 1967; Kanner 1949). These theories did not explain the aetiology of the condition and have been out of favour for several decades. They did untold damage to families in probably encouraging nondisclosure for fear of mothers being labelled defective parents.

There is a valuable lesson here and that is the need for caution when attributing *intentionality* to those with autistic spectrum disorders. One cannot assume that the motive attributable to a typical person is apposite for someone with AS even when the external behaviours appear similar. For instance, someone with AS may appear rude in conversation, due to candid comments, while not intending to be rude. A typical peer may intend to be rude by using similar comments to humiliate another. Wide discrepancies in motives for dissimilar behaviours are also in evidence.

Two groups of adolescents, one typical and one with AS, were questioned about loaning money to another peer who was unfamiliar to them. The unfamiliar peer had lost his bus fare but identified himself as a new person in the same school and promised to repay the money the next day. Of the typical peers, five out of six stated they would loan the bus fare as: (a) it was a small amount of money, and (b) they would know how to 'read' him. The six AS adolescents would not part with the fare because: (a) they were dealing with a stranger; (b) he probably would not repay the fare; (c) he would think he had found a 'sucker' and ask for more money; and (d) he might be a drug addict.

Understanding the mindset

We begin with an extreme example of the style of thinking and behaviour of some of those with AS.

Jim and Tom were adult males with AS. They moved from a hostel to independent accommodation that was monitored by a careworker. One evening the careworker decided that television access would be restricted – in the interest of furthering interaction – and removed the remote control. Jim immediately ran to the kitchen to get a knife, necessitating the careworker to take refuge in a study and barricade the door. Tom began kicking down the door. The careworker quickly offered to return the remote control. This calmed the situation and the aggrieved parties settled down to watching the television again. Understandably, the careworker did not return to supervisory duties for quite some time.

We draw attention to this case here for one simple reason. It emerged subsequently that the careworker had almost no grasp of the implications of having Asperger syndrome. What the well-intentioned careworker believed was a reasonable intervention in other circumstances was extremely inflammatory in this case.

At a conference on AS, attended mainly by adults with AS and their families, a young psychologist was amazed by the behaviour of people at the tea/coffee breaks. The tea and coffee dispensers were at the end of a ten-metre bench. From time to time, attendees (mainly with AS) approaching the bench enquired loudly, 'Where is the tea?' or 'Is that coffee? I hate that.' 'Where is the tea?' The psychologist was amazed by the amount of 'rudeness' she witnessed. Despite her expectations, feedback after the conference was very positive, although a minority complained in great detail about either a shortage of milk, teas, coffee or even the biscuits not being of the 'oatmeal' variety.

Therapists new to Asperger syndrome may form the impression that the syndrome is rooted in deep cynicism about the world. Their first encounters with a negative social outlook are often unsettling. It is a fact that people with AS can initially present as cynical, difficult or truculent. The therapeutic challenge is to overcome resistance through finding a footing in the worldview of those with AS. The worldview of someone with AS is not easily unpicked without understanding the person with AS relative to other peers. In a school setting, this means getting reports from teachers, and obviously parents. Third party reports on routines, areas of rigidity, level of concrete explanation expected and so forth are crucial to grasping the nature of AS before any intervention can occur. The absence of biological markers for the condition places an increased burden on mental health professionals to pay close attention to almost every behavioural nuance and detail. In order to contextualise and make sense of these observations, some knowledge of the various theories and hypotheses about autistic spectrum disorders (ASDs) is essential.

Current theories of ASDs have drawn heavily from various banks in the philosophy of mind and language. Mental health professionals are usually surprised to hear this, and even perplexed, but it is an incontrovertible fact. Most of what we now identify as modern science began one way or another in philosophical speculations about the nature of causality, matter and transformation. The profound differences between the autistic mindset and the typical mind are philosophical gold in their importance.

The imprecision and vagueness surrounding the biology and neural base of the condition encourages plural explanatory efforts. In the case of classical autism early clinical diagnosis is somewhat easier to achieve. Those with AS, however, are often diagnosed much later than those with 'obvious' developmental delays. Usually, a referral for diagnosis is prompted by school or parental concerns about social interaction difficulties. Many are diagnosed either late in primary level education or early in secondary level. Indeed the co-occurrence of psychiatric disorders in adolescents can make it difficult easily to diagnose AS or an autistic spectrum disorder (e.g. depression, anxiety disorders, attention deficit hyperactivity disorders, ADHD, adjustment disorders, and more; see Chapter 7).

Emerging neuroscientific explanations have implicated many areas of the brain associated with language, emotion and planning. The search for explanatory neuroscientific models for the condition is of pressing importance. Most studies now adopt the hypothesis that ASDs are not localised to a particular part of the brain but are either diffused due to connectivity problems between various brain components, or else make use of atypical pathways to process and act on information. Facial recognition, especially the recognition of emotional expression, has received a great deal of attention (Etkin *et al.* 2004; Yovel and Kanwisher 2004). Studies have produced uneven results (Boucher, Lewis and Collis 1998; Carver, Dawson and Correspondence 2002; Hadjikhani *et al.* 2004; Klin *et al.* 1999; Valdizan *et al.* 2003). Children with classical autism and some of those with AS experience a variety of difficulties fitting faces to familiar voices, recognising faces of caregivers with some not discriminating between orientation of faces (right side up or upside down). It is no wonder that, compared to their peers, many young people with AS find recognition of facial expressions very challenging.

We discuss these theories in order of historical emergence, though one could argue that this is also an accurate accidental ranking of their acceptance. Before unfolding these theories, it is necessary to lay them against a canvas that is accessible to most readers. The canvas we have in mind is called 'folk psychology'.

Folk psychology

Put simply folk psychology refers to the commonsense understanding that people have of each other and the world. The central principle of folk psychology is that our ordinary 'make-up' is dependent upon modifying, storing and reasoning with beliefs, desires and intentions. The main assumptions are that people have beliefs about the world, that they entertain desires about objects in the world, and that to achieve their desires they identify goals and intentions and enact a plan.

Folk psychology is, if you like, the ordinary psychology of the 'street'. It is the vernacular expression of reason and behaviour that humans encounter everyday. It is their main frame of reference for *explaining* and *predicting* the behaviour of others. Commonly one hears someone say after an encounter with another person, 'She didn't say it… but I know what she was really thinking.' This implies a 'gap' between what was said or exhibited as behaviour, and the judgement reached by the speaker. Often, what someone else is thinking is conveyed to us by his or her actions. If someone is cooking something in a pan, we may reasonably infer that food is being prepared because someone is hungry or it is near mealtime. The human capacity to figure out what someone else is thinking, desiring or intending is quite remarkable. It is partly dependent on assessing body language or nonverbal communication, and rarely made explicit. Analysing this capacity in terms of folk psychology is one way of accessing issues in *mind-reading* that have come to play an important role in understanding ASD deficits.

The primary concepts used in discussing the processes that characterise mind-reading are beliefs, desires and intentions (BDI). Despite 3000 years of philosophy, two centuries of psychology, a century of neurological research and 40 years of brain scanning, definitions, expressions and roles for these concepts remain stubbornly contentious. This does not point to obduracy on behalf of the research communities, but more towards the profoundly complex nature of BDI in human existence. Despite disputes over frameworks, on the whole, researchers agree that whatever processes account for the acquisition of BDI, the processes 'kick in' very early in infant development (Bartsch and Wellman 1995; Gopnik and Meltzoff 1998; Nichols and Stich 2003). One of the uncontested empirical facts is that impaired manifestation of these processes could explain many of the autistic deficits in social interaction.

Theory of Mind

Autistic aloofness has come to symbolise the separateness of the autistic person from his or her peers. The aloofness seems to be combined with a diminished awareness of other people. Does this imply that the mind of someone with an ASD is very different from that of typical peers? How can we make sense of this type of question?

The guiding principle of Theory of Mind (ToM) research is that children with autism lack the ability to attribute mental states to other people (Baron-Cohen 1995). They fail to appreciate that other people have intentions, thoughts and desires. There are several versions of ToM theories, each emphasising a variation in components rather than a sacrifice of overall allegiance to the guiding principle. The use of the phrase 'theory of mind' arose first in a study of primate capacities to allegedly attribute mental states to others (Premack and Woodruff 1978). Some commentators argued that this criterion of mental state attribution was too thin to support a theory of mind that could be applied to humans (Dennett 1978). As it stood, the theory might not sufficiently discriminate the attribution of mental states from the attribution of behaviours. Dennett argued that the detection of another's intentionality, especially the intention to deceive, was a crucial criterion for an adequate theory of mind. Being able to attribute mental states to others was necessary, it seemed, but not sufficient to ground ToM. The possession of a ToM has to serve a purpose. If ToM is an innate capacity, it would be of little use if it did not affect something purposeful. ToM is significant because people use it to predict others' behaviours. The attribution of mental states, mental representations, are required to understand and predict the behaviour of others. Without humans regularly exercising a ToM, we would be blind to the motives of others.

If a child misattributes mental states, then he or she will fail to predict the relevant behaviours of others. For example, in a male version of the Sally Ann false-belief test, mental attribution skills are tested below.

1. A child Alan is looking at two other children in a classroom. One child James puts his book at his bag before going to lunch. His friend Peter sees this is happening. He sneaks over and places the book in a box. James returns. Alan knows the book is in the box.

2. If Alan were asked where James would look for his book after lunch, he would point at his bag. Alan knows that James's belief is false. Alan also knows that his view of the world is different to James's view.

3. When asked where James would look for his book, if Alan indicated that he would look in the box, Alan would be: (a) wrong, (b) not able to understand that James could have a false belief, (c) *misattributing* his own belief to James which James could not possibly share, and (d) demonstrating difficulty with mind-reading, described by Baron-Cohen as mind blindness.

Anecdotally, many parents have stories about their child having a tantrum because something he or she knew was not acted on by the parents.

> One parent reported being hit over the head with a computer keyboard by his adolescent son with AS. This was due to an internet connection problem experienced by the boy. Since both son and father were in the study at the same time, the son was angry that his father 'couldn't see his difficulty'. He was enraged that his father could sit there 'knowing' he was having a problem and do nothing. The boy had no awareness that he hadn't actually told his father that he was having problems with the computer and that his father was in fact watching TV at the time. People with AS, despite their abilities, often have trouble grasping that other people do not share their thoughts.

The ToM-derived mind blindness hypothesis has been exceptionally influential in autism research and developmental psychology for three main reasons:

1. ToM defined a research paradigm that supported experimentally testable hypotheses. One of its first successes was to show that in

the main young children with autism would fail the false-belief attribution tests when compared with matched typical children. The specificity of the ToM theory of autism accounted for a large class of deficits while at the same time leaving intact other functions. It served to delimit areas of autistic thinking and experience.

2.   ToM was an explicitly cognitive theory of the developing mind. Children formed representations of the world and others and used these to predict the behaviours of others.

3.   ToM implicitly appeals to attempts to account formally for mental processing.

The above potted version of ToM theorising (the literature grows voluminously year by year) provides enough of the scaffolding to make a reasonable stab at teasing out several intervention implications. The first point is that studies on the developmental origins of a theory of mind may be immensely significant in time. The choice of the term 'theory' in Theory of Mind implies that mental states, their contents and attributions have a systematic linkage that allows the prediction of others' behaviour. Predictions may be wrong at times, but if ToM holds value, then predicting others' behaviour is an *endowment* – biological and partly social. The manifestation of the theory, it is argued through the folk psychology of belief–desire–intention, daily tests its reliability. The existence of a ToM module in the brain (ToMM) which represents attribution information is another possibility (Leslie 1994). However, to date experimental attempts to 'locate' ToMM in the brain are at best inconclusive. We are a long way away from replacing talk of beliefs, desires and intentions with an equivalent set of neural terms.

A difficulty arises when we ask what does a theory of mind reveal about the self and subjectivity. One argument is based on circularity. We use the theory of beliefs and desires to infer beliefs and desires in others, but then reapply the same concepts to justify the theory. Peter Hobson argues that we 'use' ToM to predict behaviours and then use the explanation of the success of these predictions to validate the theory in the first place (Hobson 1995). The question is where do the basic ToM concepts come from in the first place?

Hobson implies that the debate is muddled because concepts such as subjectivity are incommensurable with ToM ascriptions of BDI. This does not imply that ToM theories are ruinously deficient, but it suggests they are incomplete. ToM may bring some clarity to framing the questions, but it does not explain the drive to interpersonal social processing that humans continuously exhibit. The use of ToM is predicated on the pre-existence of something else that facilitates the acquisition of ToM ascription skills. While few doubt that

ToM has many explanatory merits there are several central areas of human experience that it fails to address. The most important of these are communication, emotion, social interactions and socio-emotional processing.

The success of false-belief testing with young autistic children is replicated unevenly in those with Asperger syndrome (Bowler 1992; Dahlgren and Trillingsgaard 1996). Additionally, theory of mind does not account for the inability to learn social conventions in otherwise high-functioning individuals (Bauminger and Kasarl 1999; Frith 2004; Kaland et al. 2002; Klin 2000). Despite any threshold on the empirical applicability of false-belief tests, the impact of the ToM framework for approaching the understanding of ASDs is undeniable.

Central Coherence

The notion that ASDs result from an information-processing deficit is articulated in the theory of Central Coherence. The deficit relates to observed piecemeal integration of information by autistic people. It is an appealing theory as it singles out for explanation autistic fondness for detail over context, and explains it as an integrative deficit. Consequently, perseverance with tasks, routines and hobbies are possibly the result of this deficit.

Central Coherence (CC) theory is derived from work in the philosophy of language directed at teasing out the grounds for cooperative communication. One branch of this vast field, and the point of departure for CC, is *relevance theory* (Blakemore 2002; Sperber and Wilson 1995). Despite the philosophical literature, the theory is difficult to place in a developmental framework. In Baron-Cohen's words it is 'a slippery notion to define' (Baron-Cohen and Swettenham 1997).

Primarily CC is a theory about communicative relevance, though researchers have argued that it is intrinsic to the 'proper' organisation of the mind: it governs the correct inference of mental states (Frith and Happé 1994; Happé 1999). The model advanced in support of the thesis is based on information-processing insights. Coherent classification of information indicates an intact functioning mind; a mind which appreciates organisation, but not just any kind of organisation. The mind in question exhibits central coherence in its operations. Relevant pieces of information are distinguished from irrelevant. The importance of this in understanding the mind, especially the autistic mind, is that the latter frequently demonstrates irrelevant modes of operation and response. Unsurprisingly with its linguistic footing the characterisation of the mind's irrelevant wobbles is detected primarily in language use. Irrelevance in conversation, reclassified as *weak central coherence*, is revealed through off-topic responses or atypical replies to questions. Happé's *Strange Stories* test illustrates some of the thinking behind the theory (Fletcher *et al.* 1995, p.124):

> A burglar who has just robbed a shop is making his getaway. As he is running home, a policeman on his beat sees him drop his glove. He doesn't know the man is a burglar, he just wants to tell him he dropped his glove. But when the policeman shouts out to the burglar, 'Hey, you! Stop!', the burglar turns around, sees the policeman and gives himself up. He puts his hands up and admits that he did break in at the local shop. Why did the burglar do this?

A relevant response might be that the burglar believed that he had been seen by the police officer breaking in to the shop. A less relevant response might be that he thought the police officer was looking for information about another crime. While many responses are possible, the CC theory argues that only a small number will cohere with the narrative.

In scale, CC is much less grand than ToM in its ambitions. A large number of studies have shown that a mark of autistic thinking is a propensity towards giving 'offbeat' interpretations of narratives compared with typical peers. This can be interpreted in a number of ways, running from a mark of genius and non-conformity through to poor grasp of communicative conventions (Fitzgerald 2004). Weak Central Coherence (WCC) hypothesises that the autistic mind integrates information in a piecemeal fashion such that the whole is less than the sum of the parts. Hence, while a typical person might focus on general features in a cinema, the person with autism might fixate on a doorway or exit light. What we find in WCC is blindness to contextual relevance.

Undoubtedly, WCC is consistent with the pared down understanding that autistic people have of others. However, within the broader theory of mind, WCC only makes sense if CC makes sense. This implies that relevance theory itself must make sense and be convincing. Currently, opinions on relevance as a linguistic (or psycholinguistic) construct are divided. First, people respond differently to the same narrative – look at market research surveys, for instance – the context of the response is not a reliable predictor of the actual response. Differentiating between relevant and irrelevant responses may be impossible without also distinguishing between degrees of relevance (within sets of relevant responses). Second, it is not evident that WCC is anything more than episodic. It may not continuously manifest itself when presented with an opportunity. Studies by Happé, for instance, of inference and sentence ambiguity showed that individuals with autism were less likely to choose the most coherent bridging inference or to use the most coherent account of context in the tasks. These studies have not been consistently replicated (Jolliffe and

Baron-Cohen 1999; 2001). Frith originally mooted that WCC could explain ToM deficits, in the sense that ToM deficits were notionally derivable from WCC (Frith 2003). If this were true, then the existence of ToM would hinge on a pre-existent regulative coherence principle. The argument at the time was that WCC explained why social interaction failed due to an inability to extract and pull together the relevant mental state ascription cues. However, subsequent experimental work by Happé showed that even those autistic individuals with (relatively) intact ToM could equally demonstrate WCC. Hence, ToM deficits were not consistent with WCC.

One can accept that ToM in typical individuals does not explain all aspects of social understanding, without committing to WCC as an explanation. Possibly the most that CC does is filter the environment efficiently for subjective experience; for example, perhaps by way of directing attention to more salient rather than less salient features, salience being both learnt (activated) and an evolutionary inheritance. This is purely hypothetical at present. More pertinently, the question of its connection with the development of self and subjectivity is obscure. Is the CC deficit due to social cognition problems, or the reverse? This question also echoes some of Peter Hobson's concerns about the introduction of explanations of deficits abstracted away from a developmental context. It may be the case that WCC, if it makes sense, is due to autistic experiences during infancy.

From an intervention perspective, CC draws attention to piecemeal processing and tendency for unexpected responses. In this way it reminds us that all that we may think salient in the intervention may not be identified as such by participants. This is an important lesson to draw from the work. One person's saliency may be another's irrelevancy.

A brief note on brains

We are living through a time of exciting developments in brain science with research focusing on cognitive neuroscience. Internet access allows professionals and parents to keep in touch with important developments. One of the theories of autism focuses on a part of the brain called the limbic system and on a particular part of it called the amygdala. The amygdala is a small almond-shaped structure in the medial temporal lobe adjacent to the anterior portion of the hippocampus. It is known to be involved in the experiencing and processing of emotion, in memory and social responses. Studies to date have been divided between post-mortem analysis of the brains of autistic people and using the evolving neuroimaging techniques on people with ASDs performing various tasks. However, the main areas of interest are related to emotion processing, language comprehension and organisational skills.

Limbic system (amygdala) theory of autism

Despite widespread acceptance of the neurodevelopmental abnormality hypothesis, there is (as of now) no specific brain-related test for AS. Bauman and Kemper (1994) found histoanatomical abnormalities in the medial temporal lobes structures in autism. Subsequent studies at post mortem on the brains of those with ASDs are inconclusive, with no single major abnormality identified to date that could explain ASDs (Bauman and Kemper 1994; Gillberg and Coleman 2000). However, studies have linked the amygdala to socio-emotional functioning in both primates and humans, and facial recognition impairments in autism. Recognition of *social emotions* is more impaired than recognition of basic emotions such as facial expression of fear. Reduced activation of the left amygdala was noticed when implicitly processing emotional face expressions (Critchley *et al.* 2000). Similar studies of individuals with high-functioning autism and Asperger syndrome reveal less impairments recognising basic emotions from facial expressions, but similar impairments in social emotion recognition (Adolphs, Sears and Piven 2001; Grossman *et al.* 2000).

Abnormalities have been identified in the parts of the brain that play a role in memory recall and regulating emotion and fear – the hippocampus and the amygdala – but their overall significance is still subject to further elaboration (Cahill, McGaugh and Weinberger 2001; Gillberg and Coleman 2000; LeDoux 2002).

Functional neuroimaging has shown that there is a failure in autistic brains to activate the amygdala while making judgements about emotional states (Baron-Cohen *et al.* 2000). Such evidence that there is suggests that the amygdala, which is assumed to play a fundamental role in creating 'social intelligence', functions differently in people with AS than in their typical peer group (Baron-Cohen *et al.* 2000; Welchew *et al.* 2005).

Neuroplasticity

Neuroplasticity is a phrase that is entering increasingly into common usage. It refers to the theory that the brain is plastic at various developmental stages. Depending on environmental factors (and their impact on genetic factors), brain functions develop differently. More importantly, the plasticity of the brain implies that enhancements can be achieved by targeting parts of the brain with specific therapies (Robertson 2000). In the case of patients with serious brain damage, the potential for therapies tuned to neuroplasticity is of major significance. The treatment of dyslexia through neural plastic therapy is an example of the type of condition being targeted (Troia and Whitney 2003). It may indeed be the case that effective psychotherapeutic social interaction interventions may in the future be shown to impact on brain plasticity in people with AS. Currently diagnosis of AS is still based on observation and reports about the behaviours of the person under examination, mainly drawn from third parties identifying difficulties in communicating with peers, atypical interaction styles, lack of flexibility around changes in routine, limited or no interest in alternative imaginative play, and unusual perseverance with a hobby.

Executive dysfunction

Aspects of the self relating to the world rely on control of thought and action, planned execution of decisions, organised memory and management of 'contact' with others. These latter skills are generally gathered under the rubric of 'executive function' (EF). The reason why it is important to look over this theory is that ToM alone or ToM plus CC will arguably explain the presence of highly productive minds in bodies without the necessity to consider the social world of persons. Despite any flaws in EF thinking, it does at least recognise that there is more to managing the self in the world than mind-reading.

EF theory hints at something very important to human action – it is not always reactive. Executive functioning is hypothesised as necessary to allow us to step back from a situation, from the environment, in order to frame our actions, our responses. A great deal of interest has been shown in attempting to explain the non-ToM deficits in autism by restating these as instances of executive dysfunction (Martin and McDonald 2003; Ozonoff and Pennington 1991).

Early research hypothesised that EF impairment could be an explanatory theory for autism. Its original presentation was that conscious regulation of one's actions required a capacity to shift attention between aspects of the environment (Norman and Shallice 1986). Otherwise, the mind would be overwhelmed by the onus to respond to every aspect of sensory stimulation – every environmental cue would demand a behavioural response. The mind, realised in the brain, must possess a 'central executive' to sift among the various subsystems competing for attention. Numerous studies have shown that similar impairments exist in a number of conditions, mainly ADHD, possibly indicating a certain degree of overlap in some circumstances (Hill 2004).

One of the difficulties with EF is that it bundles many processes together that may be better treated separately by way of classification and effect. For example, a capacity to step back from one's environment and formulate a plan is at least a two-stage operation requiring a filtering of the phenomenal world and the exercise of some reasoning mechanism. If the latter, then planning by its very nature involves conceptualising the world in terms of what it is like now and what it might be like at some time in the future. Therefore the ability to form beliefs is logically prior to the exercise of executive functions (Carruthers 1996; Perner 1998; Perner and Lang 2000). Consequently, it is unlikely that ToM theories are reducible to EF.

The main lesson from EF is that organisation and planning are major hurdles for many with AS, especially if ADHD is also present. The EF theory reminds us to beware of the likely occurrence of problems due to attention deficit, impulsivity, sequencing of information, etc. The intervention described in this book emphasises the importance of foreknowledge and forward planning in optimising more adaptive functioning in social interactions. It draws on an understanding of executive function to help adolescents with AS to develop some logistic skills for more successful social interactions with peers.

Intersubjectivity deficit

One of the reservations about ToM theorising is that it is one side of the mind–body debate that has raged in philosophy for millennia. Apart from this rather abstract criticism it faces a number of other challenges arising out of its generality, problems explaining the multidimensionality of autism, and reliance on a specific model of human consciousness (BDI). ToM is implicitly constrained to a particular view of how beliefs, language and reasoning fit together. Belief–desire–intention theories share contentious assumptions about the ordering of the world and people interrelationships. There is also research suggesting that social deficits are developmentally in evidence prior to the development of ToM skills (Klin, Volkmar and Sparrow 1992).

One of the striking features of the accounts given above, and they are by no means complete in detail, is the absence of any consideration of the social milieu in which the mind develops. Irrespective of one's views on the merits of ToM and its compatibility with either brain modularity or trends in neuroscience, it provides little room for the mind's development in terms of an intersubjective sharing of experiences, thoughts and emotions with others. ToM researchers do not deny that the mind develops through refinement, far from it, but it is difficult to see how the ToM paradigm can accommodate and explain such development.

In Peter Hobson's opinion, the idea that children begin developing a ToM by theorising about mental states, intentions and desires is 'daft' (Hobson 2002). It is 'daft' because it sets aside the role of social experience in leading this development. Hobson argues that as development progresses a child learns about its subjective perspective, and the subjective perspectives of others. He emphasises that there is also the apprehension of a third perspective external to self and others – *reality* for want of a better term. The implication being that if ToM-derived interaction is the dominant modality in typical development, then grasping the existence of external emotion-driven processes is problematic.

In a range of studies of early infant development, Hobson identified an important role for emotion in assisting the child's mental development in forming judgements about other people and its own mind. Hobson draws on three strands from his work in developmental psychology, psychoanalysis and philosophy. The former two areas are of immense importance to his work, but here we will dwell on the insights he has drawn from his clinical practice. He makes no bones about describing much of what he does as a form of 'practical philosophy'. Hobson advances three theses in his work that are reactions against the inadequacies of other approaches, especially ToM:

1. The development of the mind is intrinsically coupled with social contact. The mind partakes in a *developmental process*. Minds develop in proximity to other minds, not in isolation.

2. The nature of this proximity to others involves emotional engagement with them. The 'tools of thought' emerge out of an emotional engagement with others.

3. This emotional engagement turns on the typical child's disposition towards or potential-to-realise the satisfaction and value in intersubjective experiences.

Hobson explores the latter to help characterise deficits in minds that go beyond ToM deficits. What makes his work more intriguing is the explicit ascent in his theories and clinical observations from talk of minds to talk of selves, subjectivity and persons.

One of the fundamental questions in developmental psychology is about how children acquire the various mind-related concepts discussed above. On the other hand, the questions are primarily about making sense of the same concepts. Are they coherent? Can they be plausibly advanced without contradiction? Can we make sense of the idea of a child's acquisition of the concept of other minds?

The traditional argument runs along the lines that we perceive bodies first and then by analogy with (or inference from) our own bodies and minds, we then attribute minds to the other bodies. This argument is widely disseminated approvingly in the debate about our knowledge of the consciousness of other people (Crick 1995; Edelman 1994). The subject is expected to infer the existence of other subjects. Our apprehension of persons is primary in early life. It is only later that we separate the person into body and mind. In the case of autism, something is awry with this process during either a perinatal or postnatal stage. What is obvious to the typical infant is the immediacy of the other, and a drive to engage with and relate to her or him through preferential attention to faces, mother's face, ability to get comfort from other, to seek eye contact and the seeking and enjoyment of joint attention, etc.

We may indeed form knowledge about other people based on belief–desire–intention attributions and inferences, but that is entirely different from grasping that they are people first. Hobson cites evidence that children respond to non-human objects much differently than they respond to humans. He postulates that the difference lies in their experience of emotions and feelings when in contact with a caregiver, for example: '…we come to think people have minds because we are involved with them' (p.251). He presents an example of an autistic teenager who was without friends. Despite a friendship skills course, role modelling and even the assistance of a befriender, the boy's situation did not improve. Why did it not work?

> What is so peculiar, and in this case so elusive about the concept of a friend? The answer is that the concept of friend cannot be defined by features that may be observed by one who stands outside and merely watches behaviour. One has to experience the kinds of sharing and arguing and competing and so on that make up friendship. Because most children experience these things, they do not find it difficult to learn the meaning of the word 'friend'. They already know the kind of thing being referred to, even though this thing is impossible to describe in terms of its physical characteristics. (Hobson 2002, pp.249–50)

Access to people requires a grasp that they also have subjective experiences. Through 'connecting' with people we access them directly as people, not as minds supervening on bodies.

How can we use Hobson's insights in an intervention with AS teenagers? One way is to elaborate his idea about intersubjectivity and constantly emphasise the expectations of others, the need to demonstrate reciprocity and concede ground to another's subjectivity in an interaction. Therefore, practising listening skills, turn taking and dialogue are ways of building up strands of intersubjective respect.

Genetic issues

It seems appropriate to conclude this brief review with a focus on family issues that can affect an intervention. The heritability of ASDs is marked. Several studies have demonstrated genetic linkages between parents and offspring with ASDs (Busceaum *et al.* 1999; Cederlund and Gillberg 2004; Charman 1999; Constantino *et al.* 2004; Dorris *et al.* 2004; Happé 1999; Korvatska *et al.* 2002; Muhle, Trentacoste and Rapin 2004; Rubenstein and Merzenich 2003). Many parents are aware of ASD traits in themselves, their spouses or their own siblings and parents. Access to the internet and information from AS support groups will also have raised their awareness of genetic factors.

Raising the issue of heritability is not taboo in the intervention but it must be introduced sensitively. From a therapeutic perspective, one has to ask the question: is there any value introducing these issues to the parents? If the therapist is to have an honest and open relationship with parents then passing allusions to heritability are unavoidable. These allusions are not only useful pieces of information that may help parents make sense of their own experiences but they also underpin a key process in this intervention. It is implicitly a form of therapy involving parents. Rarely is the AS set of traits 'just' in the adolescent. At least one parent and possibly a sibling are likely to exhibit several of the traits but not to the same degree of severity – or at least not to the degree that prevents them functioning in their employment. Since people with severe autism rarely find a partner to produce a family, visible family traits are invariably much milder than in the profoundly affected autistic person. In less debilitating versions of autism, such as Asperger syndrome, parents are likely to exhibit diluted traits.

A recent review of genetic research in autism estimated that the likelihood of a sibling of someone with an ASD developing an ASD was 10 to 60 times greater than the general rate of autism in society (Santangelo and Tsatsanis 2005). The review concluded that autism was one of the most pronounced psychiatric childhood disorders with a genetic linkage. Despite the apparent strength of genetic factors, no genetic markers are agreed as definitive, though there are strong candidates. Studies are inconsistent with some identifying as few as two genes and others as many as 15 or more. In addition, almost every chromosome has been implicated in influencing the condition.

From an intervention perspective, the studies provide evidence in support of therapy with the whole family, especially in terms of developing the communication and social interaction capacities of the adolescent with AS and generalising them. It has to be kept in mind that when AS is in some sense 'in the family', there is a scientifically grounded justification for a therapist to tailor his or her expectations of parental initiatives and involvement. As one mother of a son with AS explained:

> My husband and I both have AS. We can teach our son all about maths and academic subjects. I had some difficulties at work. I have been sent by my employer on a course about how to get on better with staff. We do not know how to teach our son about how to get on with other people.

One may suspect that a parent has an ASD, but the genetic studies lend greater scientific credence to a judgement that might otherwise be dismissed as a 'hunch'.

Conclusions

As can be seen from the above theories and hypotheses there is no simple explanation for the occurrence of AS or its symptoms. Frith has talked about the 'cognitive style' of those with ASDs as being different from the typical individual. The difficulty lies in specifying this cognitive style in terms that are coherent and accord with clinical experience. Each of the hypotheses outlined above suggests that it is reasonable to talk about autistic thinking as different along a number of dimensions; each dimension in turn being addressable within the social interaction intervention.

First, we conclude that the AS person's perception of other people's behaviours is different. The behaviour of others is not understood (classified) as one might expect. What is obvious and implicit is not so to someone with AS. Any intervention must have this insight factored into its content.

Second, the strengths of AS such as perseverance and hobby obsessions should be turned into levers to explore social interaction. This is achieved by simply asking an adolescent to give an account to his intervention group of his favourite activity or hobby and then inviting questions from the group. In this way the focus on detail becomes a link in forging a social chain.

Third, organisation and planning are often poorly executed by AS adolescents. It is well and good to cite historical role models that have had life successes with AS, but the bulk of those with AS will struggle to find a footing that allows them independent living. Emphasising AS genius, which occurs in a minority of cases, must be balanced against the scale of social challenges facing the averagely talented majority. The co-occurrence of anxiety, depressive disorders, attention deficit hyperactivity disorder (ADHD) and obsessive compulsive disorder (OCD) in many cases raise enormous barriers to independent living let alone educational success.

Finally, if one accepts the intersubjectivity deficit hypothesis – and there is scant reason to reject it – then some differentiation must be made between the AS adolescent's orientation towards and understanding of acquaintances, friends and company. Often the differentiation is revealed best in biographical writings or third party reports of AS behaviour.

Timmy was a 16-year-old boy with AS. His friends were drawn from the ranks of junior pupils usually three to four years younger. When asked to explain how he identified friends, he replied, 'I salute someone, and if they salute me back they are my friend.' Timmy's salute was an imitation of the military equivalent. His peers had long ago given up mocking his behaviour after warnings by teaching staff. However, new younger pupils in the school were unaware of this history.

Alan was a 40-year-old technical engineer. He was unmarried and had been diagnosed with AS when he was 35 due to family concerns about his social isolation. He frequently went to the pub with his workmates at the end of the week for a few drinks, but rarely played the role of conversational participant. He began attending for therapy after a protracted period of depression due to a change in job responsibilities. When explaining his social life, he said he was quite happy to be in company and sit in the pub for hours on end without joining in conversation. He emphasised that he was 'happy to be just be there listening to the others. I don't need to join in to enjoy myself'.

Gunilla Gerland (1997) in her autobiography reported being content with the company of a group of marginalised wayward adolescents purely because they afforded her an opportunity to 'hang out' with others, despite bouts of physical and sexual abuse by members of the same 'company'.

Pulling the various strands together, we can see that there is a style of autistic thinking about the self, others and the world that is quite different, unique in many ways, from that of the typical person. This difference arises out of the developmental uniqueness of the child. A child that is not oriented (or at least has a diminished orientation) towards social contact logically has a different world at his or her disposal than a normally developing child. The child with AS has different expectations of the world, and when the world fails repeatedly to meet those expectations the results become increasingly traumatic with age. The challenge for those offering support and therapy to those with AS and their families is to internalise these strands and incorporate their implications into their own interactions with the whole family. Let us conclude with one case that sums up several of the points above poignantly.

Russell was a graduate in his mid-twenties. He led a solitary social existence and had little or no contact with peers. When asked to recount his childhood, Russell had difficulty recalling it; almost as if his childhood was punctuated by amnesiac periods. He could recall playing with children in his street during his early years but then recalled that the playing stopped. Russell described this rupture as due to 'the other children playing with each other'. When he moved to secondary school as an adolescent, he again found himself without friends. When asked to explain how this came about, he replied that he assumed that the other people in his class had friends in school and outside school, and that they 'had enough friends'. When asked about his adolescent hobbies, Russell became quite animated. He described how he became an expert on all aspects of a popular role-playing game of the period which involved role playing in groups. He read copiously on the subject and visited the relevant 'trendy' bookstores to ensure he was up to date. Taken at face value it seemed contradictory that someone could become an expert in fashionable interactive adolescent activity and yet have formed no friendships of any quality.

Of course, it is precisely this last anomaly that originally drew Russell to the psychiatric services. Despite his mastery of content and strategy, in his own words he 'had never had a successful experience'. In other words, he had never played the game even once with other peers. His explanation for not having friends was based on an intellectualisation of social exclusion because friendship was in some way rooted in a quota system. Russell's interpretation of his social world strikes us as bizarre, but it allowed him to cope with exclusion – admittedly with psychiatric support during adolescence.

To date theories of the autistic spectrum support the intervention emphasis on correcting deficits in identifying the beliefs, desires and intentions in others. Help with identifying relevant aspects of social interactions and context is clearly required. The intersubjectivity deficit implies that the focus should be on learning to share experiences with peers, and helping the AS adolescent find sufficient common ground to affiliate with peers.

3 Communication and Language Issues

This chapter explores a series of communication and language themes that surface in many different speech and language interventions, as well as in conventional SST. Asperger syndrome and autism belong to a class of pervasive developmental disorders (PDD). Language impairments are detectable in the child with PDD as he or she first struggles to communicate. Approximately 40 per cent of those with PDD will remain mute, and as many as 50 per cent of those with autism will have poor or little useful language (Lord and Paul 1997). People with AS have interaction deficits that are frequently evident in their use of language and their comprehension of conversation, even as adults (Szatmari, Bartolucci and Bremner 1989).

Language delay and impaired used of language for communication are cited among the diagnostic criteria for autism of the DSM and ICD-10 (American Psychiatric Association 1994; World Health Organisation 1990). Accounting for the use of language socially is a complex task and no one scientific approach or preferred methodology dominates the field (Dobbinson, Perkins and Boucher 1998; Koning and Magill-Evans 2001; Landa *et al.* 1992; Martin and McDonald 2003; Shriberg *et al.* 2001).

The study of language usage covers four broad areas: *syntax, semantics pragmatics* and *phonetics*. First, there is the grammar or *syntax*, used by a person in constructing sentences. Grammar refers to the rules used to organise words into meaningful sequences (sentences). One central question is whether what a person says is grammatical relative to the age of his or her peers. A sentence can be syntactically correct but express nonsense; for example, 'The large brown concept tilted superficially'. Such marked syntactic peculiarities are not usually found in AS.

Semantics, the second area, is concerned with understanding how meaning arises when words are connected together to form sentences. Semantics is best understood as what we need to know about language to extract the literal meaning of a sentence. Semantic defects, problems with meaning, are more common in AS. Mainly these take two forms:

- expressing what one intends to convey, i.e. expressing oneself in speech or writing, accurately and intelligibly

- understanding what is conveyed by others, i.e. interpreting others' speech or text accurately, including written texts.

Taking the first case for the moment, a number of studies have highlighted problems with 'meaning' expression in conversation (Bishop *et al.* 2000; Dobbinson *et al.* 1998; Hadwin *et al.* 1997). Other studies have drawn attention to narrative comprehension and general conversation management problems (Adams *et al.* 2002; Baltaxe 1977; Bara, Bosco and Bucciarelli 1999; Bara, Bucciarelli and Colle 2001; Baron-Cohen 1988; Bishop 1997; Bishop and Norbury 2002; Frith 1989; Hatton 1998; Landa *et al.* 1991, 1992; Martin and McDonald 2004; Trillingsgaard 1999).

The third area of interest is *pragmatics,* which has to do with how we use language to communicate primarily through speech – the social employment of language. It would be difficult to offer a definition of pragmatics that would satisfy all schools of thought on the subject. There is agreement that pragmatics relates to understanding how groups of sentences are used in a social context. Broadly speaking pragmatics is concerned with how meaning is constructed through linguistically mediated social interactions. Jokes, nuances and turns of phases are understood differently at different developmental phases. For example, a child is more likely to understand 'Stop pulling my leg' as an instruction rather than a request to tell the truth, stop joking or messing around. Pragmatics also includes the study of how conversations are assembled – what are the conditions for an effective conversation. By way of illustration, here are two examples of exchanges between two typical adolescents and two adolescents with AS.

Peer 1: Did you see the film last night?	AS1: Did you watch that movie about sharks last night?
Peer 2: Yeah, it was great. Did you?	AS2: Yes.

The typical adolescent exchange provided for topic maintenance. The film can continue as the focus of the conversation until one of them signals he wants to introduce a new topic. The AS adolescent exchange appears to preclude this option – if one interprets it according to the *normal* rules for discourse. However, the boundary between semantics and pragmatics is not sharp. At least half the studies cited above also reference both semantic and social language usage deficits. A common pragmatic deficit in AS is adherence to literal meaning. It impinges directly on the quality of social interactions with peers, since peers are likely to use indirect meaning frequently. Misunderstanding indirect meaning, pragmatic meaning, is an indicator of awkwardness among peers.

The fourth area of interest is *phonology*. It describes how the sounds are realised in words and in turn how this process comes to be realised in language (more properly its grammar). Spoken words are constructed from phonemes. These correspond approximately to syllables. Understanding spoken conversation is dependent upon our ability to segment sequences of sounds into sentences and sentences into words. Accurate articulation of words is very important to making oneself understood. Segmental deficits are not normally associated with AS but are present in classical autism. The rhythms and patterns of sounds we use in speech enhance whatever message we want to get across. These features are known as suprasegmental properties of an utterance – prosody. The use of sound modulation lends prosodic shape to our utterances. There is a world of difference between quietly whispering 'Open the door please' and shouting the same sentence when a building is on fire. The former conveys no sense of urgency unlike the latter. Prosody is a source of difficulty for many people with AS. Prosodic deficits are most obvious in a monotone delivery of information. There is a complex and dynamic interrelationship between a social context, the words used, and their vocal expression. Adolescents with AS struggle to get any purchase on the rules and are quickly isolated as a result by peers.

Traditionally, the analysis of conversation draws on sources in linguistics, philosophy and psychology. The study of language in spoken communication is usually referred to as conversation analysis or discourse interpretation. It embraces both pragmatics and phonology. There are many different and conflicting approaches to studying conversation, but our task does not require reviewing the various theories. The approaches roughly divide into three categories: *normative, quantitative* and *qualitative*.

Normative approaches assume that conversation is well ordered due to constraints and rules that can be stated in quasi-mathematical models (Asher and Lascarides 2003). The advantage of this type of approach is that language features can be stated and modelled rigorously. A major disadvantage is the awkward fact that many conversations are often less well ordered and predict-able than assumed, yet we muddle through. Disorderly features of conversation are either not satisfactorily explained by the models or else ruled out of bounds. *Quantitative* approaches concentrate on identifying features of conversation without necessarily worrying about whether they fit one abstract model or another. The focus is on identifying measurable features of language usage (Shriberg *et al.* 2001; Tager-Flusberg 1995). Properties of speech and frequency of word or phrase use are typical sources of interest. In contrast, *qualitative* analysis concentrates on examples of how actual conversation participants manage their conversations. It does not seek a grand theory but attempts to identify how features identified in studies are deployed in practice (Dobbinson *et al.* 1998; Koning and Magill-Evans 2001; Landa 2000; Landa *et al.* 1992). The crucial question is how robust are the results from quantitative analysis? Casual conversation poses acute challenges to many theoretical frameworks, (Eggins and Slade 1997). Yet in practice, casual conversation is the stuff that helps us define and maintain our social world. It is at the heart of satisfactory social experiences. In conclusion, what we learn from various competing approaches is that there is general agreement on gross features of conversational impairment but analyses differ widely.

Martin and McDonald (2003) observe that one of the great downsides of current research into pragmatic impairments is the lack of cross-referencing among the various theoretical positions. They also identify a bias in autistic spectrum disorder studies towards understanding language comprehension rather than language production, when in practice both comprehension and production are important. Analysing the likelihood of Theory of Mind (ToM), Weak Central Coherence (WCC), and executive function (EF) accounting for pragmatic deficits, they conclude that is it impossible currently to identify which is most suitable. The problem is that current theories can be extrapolated to make overlapping predictions. Since they all appear to offer a tentative explana-tion of a deficit (failure to grasp sarcasm, for instance), there is no reason to favour one over another, or any of them when it comes to understanding the causes of pragmatic impairments.

Returning to autism, most of the pragmatic impairments appear early in childhood after speech is first used (Parisse 1999). Mastery of vocabulary varies across the autistic spectrum. AS children often use an 'adult' vocabulary more than their peers. Prosodic deficits are common. They may speak with a monotone pitch or a very formal 'stiff' tone that persists into adolescence and beyond. Their voice modulation affects communication success. All of the diffi-culties cited above affect social interactions, producing negative outcomes and heightening awareness of exclusion, (Bjorn, Gillberg and Hagberg 1999;

Blacher *et al.* 2003; Engstrom, Engstrom and Emilsson 2003; Gilchrist *et al.* 2001; Molloy and Latika 2004; Szatmari *et al.* 1989).

Pragmatic capacities: learning from language studies

The primary weight of the intervention is on improving AS adolescents' social interactions with peers. While research studies are immensely important to progress understanding, they are riddled with different theoretical perspectives and methodologies. As a result, it is difficult to identify their implications for interventions without seeming to entertain one theoretical bias over another. This is unavoidable given the partial knowledge we have about autism and Asperger syndrome. Adopting a qualitative approach seems most feasible. First, there is an emphasis on understanding how people actually manage conversation. Second, as mentioned earlier most research has focused on language comprehension in autism rather than language production. Third, and as a corollary, isolation, loneliness and peer rejection are major contributory factors to the development of long-term suffering in the AS adolescent. These take the form of anxiety disorders, lowered self-esteem, depressive illness, suicidal ideation and alienating behaviours. Reducing the risk of social exclusion is related to the frequency of satisfactory peer interaction and this entails socially appropriate use of language. Learning to say the 'right thing' in the 'right context' contributes to the mental well-being of the adolescent. Developing positive social attitudes is a major challenge. Due to the genetic linkage between parent and offspring, parental communication patterns are also of major interest. Encouraging parents to use constructive positive comment at all times, rather than reinforcing negative social comment so frequently expressed by the AS adolescent, is an important task.

The approach favoured in this intervention is highly dependent upon dialogue, reasoned persuasion and practice with the participants about the basic requirements for peer interaction. Through these methods, we develop and enhance the pragmatic *capacities* of the participants. We use the broad notion of capacities rather than a thin one of *skills* to signal the inclusion of cognitive, behavioural and emotional components. The capacities of interest include the following (Dobbinson *et al.* 1998; Eggins and Slade 1997; Grice 1975):

- topic introduction
- topic maintenance
- repairing misunderstandings
- using acknowledgement and go-ahead signals

- avoiding repetitiveness

- controlling interruption

- understanding turn-taking dynamics.

These *pragmatic capacities* refer to a range of judgements, processes and skills that people typically draw upon when using language for communicative purposes. They include prosodic skills, which 'layer' an utterance with important emotional information.

In ordinary life, we take for granted an understanding of the conventions underpinning language usage. For example, you are in a café and need sugar for your latté but the nearest bowl is on an adjacent table. You might think it odd if having asked a customer at the table to pass you the sugar that she replied affirmatively but did not pass the sugar.

'Could you pass the sugar please?' you enquire politely.

'Yes, I could' replies the customer as she continues reading her magazine.

What has happened here? Well, in simple terms the customer has understood your request literally as a query about her physical ability to give you the sugar bowl. She has replied honestly that indeed she does have the physical wherewithal to pass the bowl. Of course, you did not *intend* to enquire about her physical capacity to pass the bowl, you *intended to convey* that you would like the sugar bowl and *expect* her to pass it over. The key point to remember here is that you tried to convey your intention to her (*the sugar please*) and your expectation (*she will pass it over*). Whatever the reason, she failed to grasp the intended meaning. She has replied to the literal meaning of your question. What strikes a typical speaker as odd about this exchange is not that we have conventions around using cafés, lattés and sugar bowls but that we have conventions around making requests of others. In this example, the other customer does not seem aware of these conventions.

Conventions, implicit rules, govern the use of language for social purposes in social settings. A vast range of implicit rules and nuances help us communicate effectively – especially in social settings. A footing in pragmatics is therefore a prerequisite for successful social interactions.

Conversational routines: communicating with others

What a sentence literally means may be worlds away from what we intend to say. For example, you see a person being detained for shoplifting and comment to a friend, 'He'd be a nice dinner guest.' Of course, what you mean is the exact opposite to the literal meaning. You are relying on your friend's grasp of the context, knowledge of your beliefs and values, and familiarity with sarcasm. People with AS find sarcasm and departure from literal meaning bothersome and troubling. Indirect meaning is confusing to them.

> Bill (13 years) enquired about hanging up his coat. He was told to 'throw it over the back of the chair'. Bill was outraged that anyone would suggest he 'throw' his clothes about. When Eileen (13) was asked to 'move desks' in her class, she tried to physically move her desk to the designated position, rather than simply swap seats. Thomas (14) found the discussion of animals in biology highly confusing. He had classified them into omnivores, carnivores and herbivores, and constantly asked for clarification on the category of animal under discussion.

In the instances above, requests and terms that are commonly used in ordinary language proved perplexing. Other acute instances involve the use of idiomatic phrases used to feign shock or surprise. It is quite common for adolescents to use 'their own' idiomatic expressions, for example, far out, awesome, savage, get out of it, etc.

> When questioned about being out of school Colin (15) said that he was 'sickened' by the other boys' conversations. He especially disliked them exclaiming 'savage' to indicate their satisfaction with a movie, computer game or music CD. 'They sound so stupid and immature,' he said. He could not bring himself to use idiomatic phrases unless they related (to his liking) in a concrete or logical fashion to the object being commented upon.

This disapproval of peer communication patterns and preferences is quite common. Unfortunately, peers identify it as arrogant and dismissive, leading to friction and bullying. Whereas the person with AS might express scepticism about a peer's claim with a direct retort ('I don't believe that happened'), typical peers might blunt their comments idiomatically ('get out of it', 'you're having me on', etc.). It is not easy to teach the use of idiomatic responses to those with AS. The appropriateness of an idiomatic response relates to both the context and the audience. Misjudging either is likely to produce embarrassment and invite ridicule.

There are a number of reasons for focusing some attention on idiomatic expressions at this stage. First, adolescents use such expressions freely. They take these expressions for granted – as part of the conversational scaffolding. Second, impaired comprehension and usage of these type of expressions immediately singles out a peer as very different from the group. Third, part of the development of a social identity in adolescence (and exploration of independence) involves experimenting with what we broadly term 'youth culture lingo'. At times, AS adolescents encounter great hardship with this very same culture. A therapist can help a group make a list of the most perplexing (and irritating).

Many less puzzling phrases can also cause comprehension and usage problems. One common instance where literal meaning is overridden by specialised phrases involves the use of conversational routines (Aijmer 1996). These routines amend the literal meaning of their associated phrases, for example:

- Honestly...

- Let us face facts...

- At the end of the day...

- To be absolutely honest...

- Stop me if I am too boring...

- I don't mean to intrude but...

- No matter what way you look at it...

Usually, the expressions signal to the hearer that what follows may be to the point, blunt, indiscreet or somewhat uncomfortable to hear. The expressions mark points in the conversation where a shift will occur. In the literature, similar phrases are termed *discourse markers*. In the intervention, we extend this definition to cover AS needs, naming them 'stock phrases'. The AS group is encouraged to practise these stock phrases to master participation in short conversations with peers.

Other entrenched routines have roles that are more transparent. These expressions relate to the proper exhibition of a range of acts associated with the following:

1.   *Apologising* ('Sorry about that …'): What is required here?

   • Recognise that something has occurred.

   • Whatever occurred caused offence to someone else.

   • Accept responsibility for what has occurred and its impact on others (e.g. 'I am sorry I scratched your CD. Can I replace it?').

2.   *Complimenting* ('I like that…'): What is required here?

   • Identify the person to compliment (i.e. look at them).

   • Identify the object of the compliment (e.g. dress, music, exam result).

   • Make the compliment using a positive qualifier (e.g. 'I like that dress', 'good music', 'great exam result', etc.).

3.   *Greeting* ('Nice to see you…'): What is required here?

   • Identify the person to greet.

   • Make eye contact (check that it is returned).

   • Make the appropriate verbal or nonverbal gesture ('Nice to see you', 'How are you doing?' or wave).

4.   *Thanking* ('I appreciate that…'): What is required here?

   • Acknowledgement of another's act that was appropriate (e.g. receiving service in a shop, accepting food at home, expressing appreciation for the action of a peer, etc.).

   • Make eye contact.

   • Make the appropriate verbal response (e.g. 'Thank you', 'I appreciated that meal', 'It was good of you to help me with the homework', etc.)

Many of these acts require the exercise of a formula – a rule or set of rules. Some of these are so trivial at one level that a therapist may be surprised that they have not been internalised: for instance: 'I like your computer screen' is preferable to 'I am disposed towards your choice of computer monitor.' One might be tempted to gloss over these conversational formulas as mildly interesting, but they cause profound difficulties for many people with Asperger syndrome.

A common question asked by many therapists and parents is whether a list of such acts could be assembled, and if so where could they get a list. This is quite a reasonable request but it misses the point. Knowing a routine and being able to use it effectively are quite separate abilities. Reading books on carpentry does not qualify anyone as a carpenter. At a certain point in time, one has to stop buying carpentry books and pick up the tools to build a box. Unless the intellectual carpenter tries his hand at a few practical projects, his knowledge is sterile. The second comment is that people do not learn to interact successfully by learning voluminous lists of formulas. They learn by adapting earlier successful formulas to context. The final point is that no matter how many books one reads, the problem is that the real world has usually not read the same books. Adaptive thinking and planning are crucial to social interactions.

The *fluency* of social interaction is influenced by formulas like those above. Their very banality lends them their influence. The AS propensity towards concrete interpretation and literalism means that all idiomatic expressions are potential obstacles – even the most obvious to the typical peer. The production of speech in conversation that is fluent and coherent, and possesses an idiomatic naturalness is a major challenge facing the AS adolescent. Unsurprisingly, the diagnostic categories for Asperger syndrome specifically mention tendencies towards odd prosody and pedantic speech patterns.

By way of illustration, it is quite common for parents to report that their son (or daughter) has been repeatedly told by peers to 'shut up', 'stop talking' or 'stay on message'. These reactions by peers indicate that the AS adolescents' contributions are not 'fitting in' on probably many different levels.

Dara was a 14-year-old boy with AS. He had repeated negative encounters with schoolmates. These encounters involved some form of bullying and ridicule. As a result, he became severely depressed and was threatening self-harm. His parents removed him from the school temporarily. Investigations by the school authorities revealed that he was perceived by peers as (a) interrupting conversations with contributions unrelated to the topic at hand; (b) intruding into the private space of others at lunchtime by following them around; and (c) had as a hobby the history of the Old Testament (the Hebrew Tanakh) which he talked about at great length if given the slightest opportunity. His peers further described him as 'not listening' and 'not interested in what guys talk about'. He also 'stared' at others when they were in conversation. The school responded by more closely monitoring his movements and steering him away from potentially troubling encounters.

Dara's experiences are far from unique for adolescents with AS. He had profound difficulties with active listening, initiation, sequencing, topic shifting and turn taking. Compounding these problems was his poor grasp of pragmatics involving idioms and nuances. Again, these go right to the heart of the communication deficits in Asperger syndrome.

> Peter was 12 years old when he came to the attention of the mental health services. He had great difficulties interacting with peers. His teacher at the time described him as antagonistic and sometimes spiteful. He would frequently correct both his peers and teacher if he believed them to be in error. His corrections could result in tantrums if they went unheeded. It was strangely ironic that he had an almost paralysing difficulty writing anything himself. He would spend hours checking and rechecking the punctuation in even a brief paragraph. He rarely initiated conversation with peers. When he was drawn into class conversation, his contributions were either vague or disparaging. He spoke slowly with none of the fluency of his peers. He had little interest in the banter between his classmates. Due to a combination of bullying and time out of school, his parents sought professional assistance. Peter was diagnosed with AS and obsessive compulsive disorder.

We see again in the case of Peter just how important it is to have a grasp of the basic conventions governing communication in social interactions. Haranguing peers over their mistakes is not an effective friendship strategy. Even though Peter was young, he did not understand that communication serves many purposes, one of them being the gathering together of peers that are not hostile. He also did not understand that his conversational routines had an impact on others, with consequences for himself. The connection between social interaction and conversational rituals runs deep in human society. The importance of ritual in human interactions as a force for improving social and affective bonds has been explored in several studies by anthropologist Erving Goffman (1971, 1981, 1982). These are precisely the bonds that cause problems for those with AS.

It seems increasingly clear from both research and biographical writings that people with AS either cannot or do not recognise the ritual nature of much of everyday communication and social interaction. For instance, asking someone how they are, making casual conversation, or complying with requests often seem pointless to people with AS. Why bother with politeness at all is a likely refrain. They fail to recognise that mutual support can be achieved from following these rituals. A number of writers with autistic spectrum disorders have explicitly commented on their puzzlement when witnessing various ordinary interaction rituals (Gerland 1997; Grandin and Scariano 1986; Holliday Willey 1999). These rituals range from greeting someone to the behaviour of people in distress due to disappointment.

At a more profound level, as argued in the previous chapter, they have no cognisance of the value of mutual support, of *intersubjective* relations with others (Hobson 1995, 2002). Here intersubjectivity involves sharing in the feelings and thoughts of others. Hobson characterises this as a major stage in human development. It is a linking of one's own personal experiences with those of another. Therefore, it underpins both reciprocity in social interaction and *empathy*. The mutuality of intersubjective linking is reinforced through rituals such as greeting, thanking, apologising, complimenting, and so on. Demonstrations of intersubjectivity are evidence of perspective taking ('stepping into another's shoes') which is arguably the basis for empathy. Taking an appropriate interest in another person's experiences and demonstrating that interest appropriately are huge areas of confusion, mystery and distress for the AS adolescent.

The fundamental tenet of this intervention is that those with AS should be taught to *treat all communication as an invitation to inference*. The message of the speaker is what is to be inferred. This message will contain meaning information, intentional information and emotional information. Coming to understand the expectations of speakers (peers) will assist greatly in extracting the message and responding appropriately. Consequently, the role played by a range of common conversational routines used by peers must be explored and practised. When a person initiates an interaction, he or she does so with the expectation that the other person (the audience) will understand what is being conveyed. The expectations that people have of each other in interpersonal interactions define the background of shared assumptions, beliefs and conventions. Socialisation, education and the inculcation of cultural practices account for the persistence of the expectations.

Individuals with AS do not apprehend these expectations as children. They do not grasp their implicit existence, social significance or permeation of all aspects of interaction. Consequently, those people are at a serious disadvantage in mundane communication settings. Even among family, ordinary social rituals may be unacknowledged.

David was an 18-year-old boy with Asperger syndrome. After a particularly protracted row at home, a consultation with his therapist was arranged. David had a history of poor social relations with peers but was academically excellent. His main relaxation was watching science and factual programmes on television. One evening his sister arrived with her boyfriend to announce their forthcoming marriage. This happened during one of David's favourite programmes. He insisted on turning up the volume and pulled his chair as close as was comfortable to the television. He neither acknowledged his sister nor her boyfriend, and eventually his father switched off the television. David stormed out of the room and spent much of the rest of the night shouting insults from the top of the stairs.

David could not set aside his perseverance with his interest to greet his sister or her boyfriend. He did not proclaim any pleasure at her news. Preoccupied with himself, he saw others at that time as a nuisance.

Greeting people who arrive into your house is a reasonably common expectation. Responding to conversational overtures is a common peer expectation. Another way to conceive of these expectations, and it does not matter if we cannot list all of them even if such an notion could make sense, is that they comprise a set of presuppositions that underlie communication and socialisation. Not all of these need be understood as linguistic in nature. They may be neurological in nature, as in the assumption that people perceive faces similarly – in AS this is not the case.

Similarly, non-linguistic behaviours such as gestures and body language postures convey information relevant to interaction settings. If one recalls the case of Dara who liked to talk at great length about his interest in the history of the Old Testament, it is evident that a range of 'go-ahead' signals were not given to him by his peers. His persistence therefore is interpreted as irritating and obtuse. Understanding the non-linguistic aspects of social interaction is extremely important to maintaining one's self-esteem.

Communication deficits in Asperger syndrome

The assessment of pragmatic skills is problematical. One qualitative approach uses a Pragmatic Rating Scale (Landa 2000; Landa *et al.* 1992). There is no doubt that pragmatic rating scales are far from being foolproof assessment instruments but they provide useful heuristic information nonetheless. Many published social skill programmes have generated their own skill checklists and a therapist may find these useful as well. Much depends on resources and the legacy of interventions already in place in an institution.

Below we produce a slightly modified version of Landa's Pragmatic Rating Scale (PRS) that we have found helpful in signalling a range of pragmatic difficulties among AS adolescents. An AS adolescent may not exhibit all the pragmatic deficits identified in the PRS, but it is convenient for annotating deficits that are displayed. The granularity of the PRS categories means that detailed profiles of communication patterns can be assembled over time for any participant. An additional objective is to use the PRS as an aid in evaluating the intervention with a particular group. A therapist can generate a scoring system using the PRS straightforwardly. Subjects with high scores in categories have difficulties demonstrating the requisite judgements and skills.

We tend to deploy the PRS over a series of conversations with the participants in the first four adolescent sessions. A similar approach should be taken with the parents. Judgements that are derived from one series of verbal exchanges may produce an unreliable rating of a participant's difficulties. A more stable rating is achieved, in our opinion, over a series of conversations.

The advantage of the PRS is that it provides therapists with a frame of reference for assessing communication capacities among those on the autistic spectrum. It is also intelligible. Along this dimension, it can be seen as a kind of yardstick that one might run over a conversation to get an idea of problems. The results have to treated with a degree of caution, however, since one is sampling a small number of conversations with a particular subject. Moreover, the sampling is not peer to peer but peer to therapist. Nevertheless, the information gleaned can be used as a foundation for assessing not only current deficits in communication, but also as a basis against which to test whether improvements have occurred over the course of the intervention.

Coaching parents in the use of the PRS as a tool for both exploring their conversation styles and those of their children is desirable but not uniformly achievable. One way to get around this problem is to interview parents periodically after sessions about their adolescents' communication styles and note their PRS-related responses.

The final caveat about the PRS is that it can be a useful tool for getting a 'rough and ready' picture of someone's pragmatic difficulties. However, due to sampling considerations its outputs should be treated cautiously and are best agreed by at least two therapists. As trust builds between the therapist and the group, participants will become more relaxed and communication will improve. Despite any ratings of improvements within group communication, the question for the therapist to probe with parents (and teachers) is whether these improvements are stable in the external world.

Pragmatic categories for assessing conversational exchanges

The Pragmatic Rating Scale (PRS) is a set of 19 categories that capture important components of the social language use of parents of autistic individuals. The development of this scale was important to settle the question as to whether:

- there really were differences between the parents of autistic individuals and the parents of typically developing children

- these differences could be measured.

Landa argues that 'the social deficits in parents, while often obvious to observers, have been difficult to define and quantify' (Landa 1992, p.245). The study found that the social language of parents of autistic children could be differentiated from parents of typical children using the PRS. It is clear from the study that the parents had similar language styles to their autistic offspring, but dissimilar styles from typical. One could infer that this result places the former group of parents on a spectrum between autism and normality. It is reasonable to conclude that the categories provide some insights into the conversational properties of people with autistic traits such as Asperger syndrome.

Table 3.1 shows the 19 features of Landa's PRS. There are 17 items which are divided into three subscales:

- Awkward/Inadequate Expression (A/IE) with five items

- Disinhibited Social Communication (DSC) with seven items

- Odd Verbal Interaction (OVI) with five items.

There are two additional items of Overly Direct and Overly Indirect styles of expression.

There were statistically significant correlations found between the features within each of the subscales. Only the features of Overly Direct and Overly Indirect were not included in the statistical analysis. This is because of the low frequency of occurrence of these features in the data.

Table 3.1 Pragmatic Rating Scale (Landa *et al.* 1992)		
A/IE	Insufficient background information	Fails to indicate clearly the specific noun phrase to which a pronoun refers; uses technical jargon that a lay person would not understand; discusses events or people without providing the background information necessary for others to understand the account.
A/IE	Vague	Accounts are general and only marginally address the enquiry. Multiple questions must be asked to obtain basic details. Despite adequate quantity of verbal output, little content is present.
A/IE	Awkward expression of ideas	Semantically inappropriate use of words or figures of speech is found. Use of stereotypical phrases during a conversation even when these do not seem to make sense in the context.
A/IE	Inadequate clarification	Failure to revise an utterance sufficiently to clear up confusion resulting from the original utterance.
A/IE	Terse	Rarely speaks unless presented with a query. Mainly offers short, unelaborated responses.

Table 3.1 continued

DCS	Overly talkative	Difficult to interrupt in speech; talks too long despite being given cues to relinquish conversational turn.
DSC	Overly candid	Expresses very personal information or makes highly critical, evaluative comments about people or situations.
DSC	Overly detailed	Provides minute details about an event or recounts technical aspects when asked a general question.
DSC	Out-of-synchrony communicative behaviour	Elaborates on insignificant aspects of another's statements rather than on main point; tangential responses; frequent and obvious misinterpretation of another's statements or queries.
DSC	Abrupt topic change	Abruptly changes topic without using typical social markers that signal the change or indicate the relevance of the off-topic information (e.g. 'This is off the subject but…' or 'That reminds me of the time when…'.
DSC	Topic preoccupation	Frequently recalls previously discussed topics without being prompted to do so where discussion of previous topic is redundant.
DSC	Confusing accounts	Disorganised presentation of information; inappropriate use or absence of cohesive devices that indicate how current information is related to previous discourse.
OVI	Overly formal or informal in manner of communicating	Uses extremely precise articulation; uncommon multisyllabic words in a casual conversation where more common words would suffice; profanity.'
OVI	Little conversational to and fro	Frequently interrupts; fails to expand or acknowledge another's statements; rarely attempts to elicit conversational participation from another.
OVI	Atypical greeting behaviour	Fails to greet or acknowledge another's greeting (e.g. averts gaze; makes insulting remarks about another's presence rather than welcoming remarks).
OVI	Odd humour	Fails to signal humorous statements or to indicate the humorous nature of utterance when humour clearly not detected by another.
OVI	Inappropriate topics	Initiates topics that are wholly unrelated to the task at hand, such as rearranging badges on clothes while requested to complete an essay.
Overly direct		Excessively blunt or straightforward in expression of opinions or instructions.
Overly indirect		Unduly veiled in expression of opinions or instructions with the result that what is intended is unclear.

The PRS provides a rich set of descriptors for application to AS conversations, but it needs to be used in conjunction with (a) the assessment of pragmatic capacities demonstrated in actual conversation management; and (b) by interpreting the absence or presence of appropriate nonverbal communication, e.g. gestures, nods, eye contact.

Understanding intentionality in conversation

The inspiration for pragmatic work in conversation including the PRS goes back to the philosopher Paul Grice (1975, 1989). He was interested in conversational *inference* and *implicature*. Together these terms can be defined as how one gets from what is said to what is meant. Implicature refers to what is intended by the speaker and inference to the meaning produced by the hearer. When there is a mismatch between what the speaker intends and what the hearer produces, then there is miscommunication. This distinction between implicature and inference is important when the literal meaning of an utterance is not the intended meaning of the speaker. As Searle (1975, p.59) says:

> The simplest cases of meaning are those in which the speaker utters a sentence and means exactly and literally what he says. In such cases the speaker intends to produce a certain illocutionary effect in the hearer, and he intends to produce this effect by getting the hearer to recognize this intention in virtue of the hearer's knowledge of the rules that govern the utterance of the sentence. But notoriously not all cases of meaning are this simple.

It is clear from language studies that it is at the level of implicature, working out what the speaker intended, that those with AS have serious difficulty. What people intend to convey in conversation is far from the surface at times. To extract their intentions, their motive and their beliefs a grasp of implicature is necessary. This is a key lesson imported into the intervention.

Not alone the words themselves but also the context and background knowledge must be taken into account to arrive at the intended meaning of an utterance. With extra contextual information, the intended meaning of these utterances in conversation is clearer for typical peers but may still pose comprehension problems for those with AS. This is because those with AS have difficulty understanding contextual cues that provide typical people with enough information to correctly interpret utterances: that is, to infer the same meaning that the speaker implied. The situation is even more problematic when the context is unfamiliar. This goes some way towards explaining why people with AS dislike changes in routine. Change in routine entails change in context.

According to Grice, a speaker's contribution to discourse is governed by four maxims. These are now known as Grice's maxims (Table 3.2).

Table 3.2 Grice's maxims (after Green and Morgan 1981)	
Quantity	Make your contribution as informative as required. Do not make your contribution more informative than is required.
Quality	Do not say what you believe to be false. Do not say that for which you lack adequate evidence.
Relation	Be relevant.
Manner	Avoid obscurity of expression. Avoid ambiguity. Be brief. Be orderly.

Unfortunately, Grice's work was primarily philosophical and he was vague about how to apply his principles in practice. There are no guidelines in his work suggesting how it could be taken into clinical practice. The PRS, by contrast, aims to support an empirical test of pragmatic ability. For those who do accept Grice's theory, there are two main criticisms. First, the maxims are too general to support detailed analysis of conversation. Second, the analysis they do allow for is purely qualitative. The PRS is a sustained attempt to develop a clinically useful model from his work.

Short lessons for interventions

Certain language difficulties can be properly addressed in an intervention. These difficulties affect the appropriate use of language socially. However, other language difficulties, stammering, odd pitch or voice tone may require external speech therapy – especially if only one member of the group has the specific challenge. Dealing with a single person's language difficulty without drawing undue attention to him in the group is a sensitive issue. For example, adolescents with a monotone voice or specific prosodic oddities may be best directed towards speech therapy while continuing with the intervention. Role playing emotion in the voice can help and is part of the intervention, but it does not receive the same attention as in a dedicated speech therapy treatment. On the other hand, if the specific language difficulty is shared by two or more in the group then the therapist must make a judgement about her capacity to respond effectively to their needs.

Michael had been diagnosed with AS at the age of eight years. He had attended speech and drama classes for three years before joining the intervention. However, he had a slow and measured delivery style that lent a leaden quality to his speech. Occasionally, he would 'put on' accents and deliver lines he had learnt in drama class. He was a good mimic of accents and voices. Despite these abilities, his self-report and verbal interactions never showed the slightest hint of these skills. Regardless of whether he was describing an unpleasant interaction with a peer or recalling a pleasant occasion, his inflection and tone did not alter. Despite these vocal limitations, Michael thoroughly enjoyed the sessions and his style was never commented upon adversely by the other participants.

Addressing Michael's vocal pitch in the group without singling him out was pursued through 'emotioneering' exercises. In these sessions, participants were asked to respond in character to various video scenarios. The second phase consisted of assisting them to respond as themselves to the scenarios. We used a scenario demonstrating an upset friend to fuel these exercises but there are endless numbers of movies that could be used instead. Insofar as is compatible with the needs of the rest of the group, we favour addressing prosodic issues in the group, even if the work is complementary to external speech therapy support.

By far and away the greatest lesson from research is the persistence of pragmatic deficits. There are no easy answers or established techniques for overcoming these challenges. Almost all tasks are obvious but require time and patience:

1.   Ensure that each participant articulates words and sentences clearly.

2.   Encourage voice modulation – no whispering or shouting.

3.   Enforce turn taking – only the person holding a specific item speaks.

4.   Push participants to produce speech – prefer production to comprehension.

5.   Explore inference and implicature – indirect meaning and intention.

6.   Practise dialogue within the group – a cycle of speak–listen–reply.

We look at putting particular strategies in place in the next chapter.

Why language is not enough: other factors to consider

However, relying on language studies alone is not sufficient to script or assess the full range of nonverbal features that occur in social interactions. An intervention has to factor in extra-linguistic features that consolidate effective social interaction. Socioemotional issues are also key qualities of our interactions. Many of these features are expressed nonverbally. People with AS have difficulties reading subtle social behaviour and cues. They will find learning the requirements to engage in and maintain interactions in different settings difficult. However, nonverbal discourse skills are crucial to the development of peer interaction skills in adolescence. A study of adolescents' valuations of communications skills found four categories that were judged particularly important for friendship (Mobbs Henry, Reed and McAlister 1995):

1.   Capacity to convey empathy during shared talk about personal difficulties.

2.   Aptitude for grasping and using figurative language, humour and slang.

3.   Utilisation of discourse skills in topic management, eye contact, tone of voice and general quality of conversational exchanges.

4.   Evidence of tact in interpersonal negotiations.

All of these areas require a grasp of social cues and behaviours – precisely the areas that are most challenging for those with AS. Understanding their difficulties means understanding what extra is needed over and above the explicit conversational capacities and pragmatic categories mentioned earlier.

A prominent review of approaches to language interventions argues that this is necessary for 'planning facilitative contexts for the acquisition of knowledge of verbal and nonverbal dimensions of conversational interactions' (Prizant, Schuler and Wetherby 1997, p.590). From a therapeutic perspective, the rationale for assessing these behaviours is to build a clearer picture of strengths and weaknesses. From an intervention perspective, knowing the assessment categories assists in guiding the intervention along certain paths. Just as the inter- vention tries to steer a group towards pragmatic capacities and away from PRS deficits, equally it must integrate its approach with broad assessment categories covering verbal and nonverbal interaction features (Ashton and Harpur 2004).

The following is an example of one qualitative assessment guide covering both verbal and nonverbal aspects of communication adapted by Prizant *et al.* (1997, p.592) from earlier work (Lapidus 1985).

Verbal discourse skills

1.   Attending

- Attends to partner
- Secures other's attention.

2. Turn taking

- Initiates greetings
- Responds to greetings
- Follows partner's turn with appropriate utterance
- Yields turn when appropriate
- Allows partner to complete turn without interrupting
- Can participate in discourse over multiple turns.

3. Initiating conversation

- Introduces/establishes conversation or topic
- Uses attention getters
- Uses comments
- Requests information
- Uses variety of strategies
- Selects appropriate topic
- Takes listener's perspective by focusing on new information
- Can discuss a variety of topics.

4. Maintaining conversation

- Acknowledges others' comments
- Questions appropriately
- Uses contingent response/comments
- Presents valid and relevant information
- Signals topic shift
- Uses repetition (echolalia) to maintain conversation
- Requests clarification
- Responds to clarification requests.

5. Breakdown and repair

- Recognises breakdown

- Requests clarification
- Responds to request for clarification.

6. Metalinguistic knowledge

- Uses/understands metaphors or idioms
- Tells/understands jokes
- Understands teasing
- Gives/understands warnings
- Gives/understands hints.

7. Sociolinguistic sensitivity

- Adjusts speaking style according to listener's age, status, sex and familiarity
- Uses politeness markers and forms
- Uses appropriate vocal volume and intonation
- Avoids socially inappropriate topics.

8. Terminates conversations appropriately

Non-verbal discourse skills

1. Uses of gestures

- Points to support language use
- Gestures for size and distance
- Does not use extraneous movements that interfere with communication.

2. Eye gaze

- Establishes eye contact prior to initiating communication
- Looks at speaker when listening
- Uses gaze checks to signal attention to speaker
- Uses gaze appropriately (duration and timing).

3. Facial expression

- Display of affect is appropriate to situation
- Does not display extraneous facial movements.

4. Use of head nods and head shakes

- To signal affirmation
- To signal denial/refusal
- To signal attention to speaker and comprehension of message.

5. Posture

- Is conducive to face–face interaction
- Stands or sits appropriately in situation.

6. Proximity

- Moves closer to initiate interaction
- Uses appropriate distance
- Moves away to terminate interaction.

7. Bodily contact

- Shakes hands appropriately
- Uses touch to secure attention
- Does not exhibit inappropriate touching during interaction.

8. Orientation

- Uses appropriate head and body orientation when seated or standing.

9. Paralanguage

- Uses appropriate features for:
  - volume
  - intonation
  - pitch
  - vocal quality
  - stress
  - rate

- Speaks fluently

- Does not produce extraneous sounds or jargon.

(Prizant *et al.* 1997)

The 'Characteristics of an Effective Communicator' (Andersen-Wood and Smith 1997, p.25), the 'Social Use of Language Questionnaire' and the 'Social Language Rating Profile' (Rinaldi 1992, p.47) are also established checklists of communication skills and abilities that could be used. It is debatable whether they should be used on their own as rating tools to test communicative or pragmatic ability. In addition, the latter two programmes are largely directed at young children rather than the adolescent. Following the advice in the work of both Gillberg and Prizant, complementary psychometric assessments are essential in all intervention programmes. Nevertheless, there are many choices.

Both Rinaldi and Prizant make a clearer distinction between the roles of listener and speaker than Landa *et al.* do in the PRS. The main lessons from the 'Communication Skills Rating Chart' (Rinaldi 1992, p.12) and the 'Assessment and Intervention Domains for Verbal and Nonverbal Discourse Skills' (Prizant *et al.* 1997, p.593) are that the results of pragmatic language studies should be augmented with:

- non-verbal aspects of communication

- explicit reflection that communication requires reciprocity

- clearer division between the role of individual as listener and role as speaker.

Prizant also distingusihes between *use* and *recognition* of language that is not made in Landa's PRS, for instance. This is the distinction between *production* and *comprehension* which we flagged earlier in the chapter. The assessment of receptive language and communicative ability requires assessing an individual's language comprehension and recording the strategies she or he uses in responding to conversational overtures (Prizant *et al.* 1997). This distinction is extremely important. For example, a failure to respond to a comment such as a sarcastic comment could be for two reasons. First, there could be a failure to understand the remark; perhaps the person does not understand the inferences and the meaning intended. Second, it is possible that the person understands the meaning but does not find the remark humorous and therefore does not give a reaction.

In terms of social interaction efficacy, this distinction is important. If the intended inference is unclear, then obviously finding a way to assist people to understand utterances of this nature is important. If, however, the person did not respond due to the fact that they did not find the remark humorous, then introducing a range of politeness strategies is the preferred option.

Conclusions

In summing up, the role of the therapist in the intervention regarding language and communication is as follows:

1.　Manage prosodic deficits as best you can.

2.　Strengthen pragmatic capacities of the group.

3.　Use the PRS to understand what the group must minimise and avoid.

4.　Ensure that discourse practice includes nonverbal components.

5.　Remember the skills must be evident in the group to be used outside it.

Tendencies towards repetitiveness, interruption and turn-taking violations must be carefully monitored. It is impossible to have any success with topic initiation, maintenance and communication repair unless these former processes are brought under control. Repetitions and unnecessary elaboration in conversation are common in AS adolescents not only in those with more pronounced autistic symptoms (Harpur, Bengtsson and Lawlor 2005). Symptoms of dysfluency are more likely to alienate peers than earn their endearment.

This may have been a difficult chapter to get through depending on the reader's background, but the details about linguistic discourse and nonverbal categories are all germane to the intervention. Each session, irrespective of theme, draws on ideas in this chapter. The therapist needs a language not only to describe the verbal space occupied by the adolescents but also a language to report on the physical attributes of the verbal and nonverbal behaviours. Social interaction is not exhausted by language alone. Extra-linguistic factors are equally important if not more so in adolescence.

In this chapter, we spent time skirting around the edges of philosophical approaches to language. This is justified given the nature of our incomplete knowledge of autistic spectrum disorders. Several prominent theories are steeped in philosophical presumptions. In the second place, the business of philosophy is making the implicit explicit. This is precisely the coinage needed to address social interaction deficits in AS. Asperger syndrome in its social manifestation is an expression of the implicit going unrecognised. To address this gap those with AS have to undertake a voyage of discovery, not unlike Temple

Grandin's comparison of herself with an anthropologist at work. In our case, we guide the voyagers on their way with a compass hybridised from many disciplines. Its cardinal point simply reads: *all interaction is an invitation to inference.*

4 Assembling an Intervention

In this chapter we pull together the conclusions and insights of the first three chapters and introduce the intervention template. We assume that the group will be managed by more than one therapist. The intervention programme outlined here is directed at adolescents (and older) with Asperger syndrome (AS) and their parents. Both parties are required. The involvement of parents in social skills interventions is advantageous (Dowrick 1986; Marcus, Kunce and Schopler 1997):

1. Parents are likely to improve the efficacy of the intervention by following through on at least some of the content for some of the time.

2. There are strong ethical arguments in favour of demonstrating sensitivity towards and respect for family values not otherwise accessible to the therapist.

3. Educating parents about their adolescent's condition helps them understand which behaviours require modification both in the adolescent and within the family.

4. The intervention can support parents while they try to adjust interfamilial behaviours and encourage peer relationships.

The design of the intervention ensures that parents operate as coaches and as their own support group. Additionally, parents are assisted and encouraged to examine their own communication styles and how these influence their adolescents' modelling of interaction conventions. Parents are taught that what is learned in the intervention must be reinforced outside of it. It is a demanding requirement but essential in the real social world. Along this dimension, the intervention can be viewed as a form of family therapy.

The adolescent group participants must meet AS criteria and (as far as is achievable) be matched for IQ and age. These suggestions are consistent with a number of evidence-based observations (Howlin 1998; Myles and Adreon 2001; Ozonoff *et al.* 2002). Matched groups are more likely to cohere. Adolescents with pronounced behavioural problems (ones that are not manageable in a group) will delay the emergence of group coherence and may need separate attention.

Candidates should be carefully screened before the intervention begins and during the first three to six weeks. What happens to those that do not fit IQ and age profile of the group? There is no convenient response to this question. Adolescents that fall outside the screening range are best served in their own matched group.

Adolescents with AS do have experiences and interests in common with their peers, but often they are unaware of these. They have a connection with an education system, the television and movies, the internet and a range of other interests. The problem is that a person with AS will talk at length about his or her special interest or hobby, whereas the typical adolescent will have a range of interests. The following are examples of special interests:

- a boy (13 years) with Asperger syndrome who persistently steered conversations towards his water sports preoccupation

- another boy (14 years) was devoted to fifth-century Babylonian history – not fourth century or sixth, just fifth century

- yet another male adolescent (15 years) could list the Allied Forces' generals involved in the European World War Two campaigns, but had no interest in the other campaigns

- again another male (16 years) had an expert knowledge of church service schedules across all denominations in his area

- a girl (16 years) had an intense interest in European international relations from 1977 onwards that involved France

- another girl (14 years) was fascinated by telephone directories and would occupy herself reading and copying the entries into a ledger.

Having a special interest is not in itself a bar to peer interaction, but the adolescent has to be taught to control how he or she avails of the special interest when in the company of peers. Self-regulation influences interactions with peers. Anxiety management, which is addressed later, is intrinsically dependent upon self-regulation abilities. A special interest or hobby is often not something they have in common with peers. In the group setting, a good deal of effort and time is put into helping participants (a) relax, (b) recognise others' interests and (c) explore common ground among themselves and with peers.

People interact socially for a variety of reasons. Among adolescents, interactions are often part of a process of affiliation – making friends. Drawing appropriate attention to oneself and paying appropriate attention to others is central to the process. A social interaction is any contact between two or more people requiring reciprocal communication – communication that is responsive to each other's inputs. This could be as minimal as greeting a phone operator, or as intense as being with a stimulating date. Reciprocal communication requires a response to an action (an utterance, a gesture, a joke, etc.) with a corresponding appropriate action. For instance, if one person announces in a distressed manner that her mother has just died, responding with 'Does that mean we'll be late for the restaurant?' is not an appropriate reciprocal comment. Reciprocity is so entrenched in everyday social interactions that we tend to be quite puzzled when it is dredged to the surface for analysis. Yet we have little difficulty recognising when an interaction has broken down due to a lack of reciprocity. Communication breakdown also occurs with language misunderstandings due to ambiguity or mistaken reference. These causes are tangentially related to reciprocal breakdown, which is a major focus of interest in this intervention.

Developing strategies for understanding and responding to reciprocal communication helps create common ground among the participants. It is important for several reasons:

1. Having objectives and experiences in common creates a series of identifiable footings for conversation and interaction. School courses and exams are helpful in this respect. Those adolescents who are not currently attending school will still have a comprehension of school structure and processes. The positive interaction experiences in the group may prepare them to return to school.

2. Identifying common ground will assist the development of age-appropriate social problem solving skills. This will become demonstrably important in role plays and practice.

3. The intervention hinges on a form of analysis which is summed up in the phrase *making the implicit explicit*. In order for this to affect the

participants' interface to the social world, probing of peer relevant mutual beliefs, knowledge and social expectations is necessary.

4.   The intervention stresses the primacy of peer communication above all else. A group with too broad an age range violates this principle. Ideally, age ranges should be 14 to 16, 15 to 17, and so forth. If the distance in age and school years is too great, then the peer-to-peer interaction emphasis and common ground that help establish these footings may be less easy to establish satisfactorily.

A primary goal of the intervention is to challenge and expand the worldview of the AS adolescent. A radical shift in perspective by the participants, a 'fracturing' of their worldview, is sought. It intentionally adopts an intellectual approach to developing social interaction capacities, supported by internal and external role play and rehearsal. The intervention attempts to change the AS classification and expectations of the social world. This cognitive restructuring (thinking about the world differently) could be understood metaphorically as the gradual replacement of one pair of lenses with another. The first set of lenses was socially unifocal. The replacement lenses are better than the first. We call them socially varifocal. However, even the new lenses cannot completely correct the deficits. The intervention is not about normalising the adolescents; rather it is about improving their capacities to interact more effectively and satisfyingly with their peers.

How important is the setting?

This is a moot question. Various resource restrictions and human limitations impinge on the selection of an appropriate setting. However, some thought to the likely stresses of using one setting over another should influence the final choice. One might argue that the physical setting is incidental to the intervention. A room is a room is a room. Detailed attention is paid to the training environment in professional athletics. Sporting failure is often attributed to inadequate training facilities. The space within which the intervention is delivered is analogous to a gym for strengthening social interactions. We argue that the intervention environment merits attention to detail. People with Asperger syndrome frequently report sensory discomfort. In many cases, for example, labels are removed from shirts and other clothes worn next to the skin. Auditory discomfort is also reported and is potentially distracting. The choice of setting for the intervention should be assessed for likely sources of auditory discomfort. Screening for sources of continual noise (traffic and air conditioning), or sudden noise (doors closing), is recommended before the intervention begins.

The physical setting for the intervention requires that (a) refreshments such as soft drinks and snacks are available to the group, and (b) that the parents can remain on the premises or nearby together in a comfortable surrounding that facilitates communication among them. A hotel is probably the best venue with a large room chosen for the first phase of the intervention, but a suitably modified institutional setting may be satisfactory. Refreshments should be placed on a table in the room out of direct sight of the group. There is no reason for anyone to leave the room during a session except to use the restroom. Adolescents often feel there is something special about going to a hotel, whilst their parents wait around in the bar or restaurant, developing their own support group in tandem. We stress that this is an important component of the programme, and should not be viewed as incidental. Parents must be prepared to bring the adolescents to the venue and remain there. One AS adolescent commented that he was quite pleased that parents had to 'hang around' as he had 'often waited for them' while shopping, or at family occasions. This sentiment was echoed by others. When delivering parent sessions, there is no requirement to bring the adolescents along.

Participants sit in a horseshoe pattern with a table for a computer and projector at the open end of the horseshoe. It is probably best to begin in a big room where the group will not feel oppressed by lack of space and proximity to other members is not an issue. A smaller room is viable once congeniality and trust develops within the group. Windows should have blinds on them and walls should be devoid of distracting posters and pictures. Everyone should be focused on each other, the therapists and the projector screen when required. Desks are not used and the requirement for note taking is minimised. It was decided early in the planning for the intervention that it should avoid the flavour of school and rote learning. Infusing the learning process with enjoyment and playfulness are major delivery objectives.

The intervention consists of approximately 26 two-hour sessions given over the course of 6 to 12 months. Delivering the sessions in blocks is also feasible, depending on resources, expectations of the group and the objectives of the therapists. However, we recommend the delivery of no more than two sessions per week. Time must be set aside for real-world practice. There is a 15-minute break for refreshments in the middle of each session. As the sessions develop, the break will become an opportunity for spontaneous conversation among the adolescents. This is a litmus test for the successful integration of members of the group. If this does not occur within four to six sessions, the therapists will have to take a more active role in encouraging conversation. The occurrence of break-time conversation indicates that the members are relaxed with one another and more significantly find the interactions enjoyable. In fact, when this routine becomes established there may be difficulties getting the group to stop interacting and return their focus to the rest of the session – a rewarding moment.

What does it hope to achieve?

The intervention seeks to effect improvements in knowledge, attitudes and skills/behaviours that AS adolescents need for mutually satisfactory peer-directed social interactions. An improvement in:

- *knowledge* would cause the AS adolescent to factor in someone else's interests while talking to them

- *attitude* entails a reduction in negative comment and an increase in positive comment – constructive comments replace oppositionality and rigid patterns of reaction (behaviour)

- *skill* might amount to the use of a greeting when meeting classmates based on an understanding of the function of such actions in interactive settings

- *complex discourse skill* would include integrating turn taking and sequencing in conversation

- *organisation* of tasks and time would amount to the participants taking more responsibility for logistical tasks: arriving on time, bringing materials, complying with requests and external practice exercise all require improvements in executive functioning

- *socio-emotional expression* including self-regulation and identification of emotion in others.

Traditionally interventions for this group of adolescents strive to inculcate 'friendship-making' skills. The underlying social presumption of these models is, arguably, that the social world divides into those who have friends and those who do not. We submit, however, that many people with AS desire *social company* rather than a collection of friends. The distinction is subtle. It does not rule out friends but it does allow for an intermediate position on the social scale that may be satisfying to many with AS and will aid them to develop friendships.

The intervention strives to provide the group with an experience of successful social interactions. For many participants, this encounter may be their first experience of successful peer interaction for months if not years. Parents also experience social success. They benefit by the support afforded to analyse and change their own communication and interaction styles. A number of parents may be unaware of the amount of negative comment they produce in the presence of their adolescents. Adolescents with AS need to encounter positive comment more frequently than most. Parents are encouraged and monitored in the use of the 'banned phrases' rule which simply states that only constructive comment will be permitted in company (see Appendix 2).

Overestimating parents' capacities to contribute to an intervention may occur. Being neutral and non-judgemental in attitude when assessing their input is required. The genetic basis of autistic spectrum disorders implies that many parents will have AS traits, largely unbeknownst to them. What a parent can 'bring' to the intervention has to be assessed in this light. There is little doubt, however, that if parents are enthusiastic about their own experiences both in sessions and socially, this will influence their attitude towards the programme and have some influence on the adolescents. Similarly, the experiences of the adolescents will influence the parents. Despite the most earnest wishes, it is unlikely that many of the adolescents will discuss with parents what takes place in their sessions. Consequently, based on their long experience, parents are left to infer if the adolescent enjoyed it; an inference that is confirmed when their son or daughter wants to return the following week.

Best practice issues: towards a template

Not every child or adolescent will be seen by an expert in autistic spectrum disorders. There is a need to build bridges between different therapies and therapist backgrounds in delivering social interaction interventions. A competent committed therapist will always adapt to the needs of participants.

Identifying best practices in socialisation training is useful but needs to be integrated with the reality of therapy settings, course content and the all-important skills of the therapist(s). A tension will always exist between ideal laboratory practices and those delivered in a mundane setting. Different components of an intervention attract their own complement of best practices. An inspiring therapist with sound pedagogical principles may overcome the limitations of meagre intervention materials or resources.

The therapist is at the root of the success of any intervention. While taking cognisance of expectations of the participants, the therapist motivates, manages and resolves conflicts in the group. The therapist facilitates understanding and development of social interaction, modelling of solutions, role play and interactions. Some value judgements are inevitable when outlining best practices for an intervention with AS adolescents. They largely reduce to a lack of consistent data about the efficacy of existing interventions. The question is less of identifying the one therapy, and more of how many can be availed of successfully. The list of methods that follows is based on a review of extant literature mentioned in Chapter 3 and clinical experience.

1. Everyone participates, and the participation of everyone must be assured and managed. Quantity is better than quality in the early phase. Encourage speech production over speech comprehension.

2. Discussions, directions, commentary and feedback should always be constructive. Promote active listening at every session. Deliver praise as incentive to participate.

3. Begin with themes that are common, e.g. asking for help. Keep the initial treatments simple. Avoid language that might cause confusion. Introduce stock phrases.

4. Explore social abilities that are empirically identified by peers as necessary for successful social interaction. Problem abilities should be ones that arise in the natural context of participants' experiences. If necessary peer questionnaires can be administered to ascertain which social cognitions and skills are best suited to the local school environment.

5. Look at discourse skills that are applicable to the participants' peer environments. Any programme should be ecologically sound and reach into the participants' school experiences. Encourage participants to take an active interest in the common cultural knowledge shared by their peers in school, e.g. movies, music and sport. Move slowly from conversation through speech into conversation with speech and nonverbal components.

6. Make sure materials are appropriate and expressible within the cultural milieu of the group. The intervention content must resonate with ordinary everyday experience. For instance, there is little point in using materials with idioms and topics that are uncommon in the society of the group; to do otherwise will cause confusion.

7. Focus on what can be achieved within the time available. The duration of the intervention limits what can be achieved. Session duration should match the concentration span of the age group. Offer additional booster sessions if possible after completion of the main intervention.

8. Exploring contingency management strategies when things go wrong should be assisted by group affirmation (applause) and individual awards. Always set concrete award goals – perhaps a meal

at the end of the intervention. In the case of AS, contingency management is hugely significant in contributing to learning self-regulation and the significance of reciprocity. It must be pursued vigorously to assist participants develop cognitions and behaviours helpful to social interaction and problem-solving strategies.

9. The therapist models solutions to social interaction difficulties, pointing out the pragmatic capacities and discourse skills required. If a situation is too arousing or upsetting for participants, the task may require simplification to reassure participants.

10. An intervention should be multimodal. This means that other parties may act as social agents in the process. For instance, parents, teachers and peers are everyday social agents. The extent to which each of the latter is to be involved is dependent upon a range of group preferences and resources.

11. Ideally, an intervention should have a broad practice base with several therapists meeting frequently to evaluate progress and discuss problems. Therapists should have regular opportunities for consultation with (or supervision by) an experienced professional who understands AS, adolescents and group dynamics. Each therapist should maintain detailed session notes recording observations. Frequent meetings will help establish parameters for content and delivery. The latter is crucial, as delivery is itself a problematical variable in interventions.

12. The group should get a sense of an alliance between the therapist and themselves in confronting their problems. Often this can only be achieved when the group becomes relaxed with the therapist and this in turn requires relaxation strategies. Humour, appropriately used, can be extremely effective in dissolving inhibitions and distorted therapist-focused cognitions. The use of humour requires prudent judgement.

13. Finally, a therapist must be able to identify each interaction as fitting into a pragmatic or discourse skill category. Adherence to structure does not diminish creativity or question tailoring of approaches. Each session must be carefully planned. Therapists should have a very good understanding of AS adolescents and enjoy working with them.

Questions relating to resources, timescale and likely group and individual needs must be well thought out prior to either adopting or recommending a social interaction intervention. A number of methodological concerns need detailed assessment. Interventions that do not have a strong emphasis on social interaction may be of limited use to adolescents, as opposed to young children for whom rote learning of micro-skills may be more effective. If parents are regularly involved, then clear allocation of responsibilities will assist in identifying their contributions to the efficacy of the intervention.

A useful historical analogy to explain the differences in emphasis and methodology is reflected in the training changes that took place when typists encountered word processors back in the early 1980s. Two approaches to training were adopted. One was known as task-based training wherein the typists were trained to do various tasks using the word-processing commands. For instance, very detailed stepping through each menu option and command was emphasised. It was shown that these typists picked up the necessary skills more quickly than a second group that were subjected to conceptual model-based training. Here a higher level overview of the word-processing software was provided, with the emphasis on grasping the larger components of the system and their interdependencies, that is, a model of the system. However, it emerged that the second group, while initially less effective, over time outperformed the former group, especially when problems arose. The latter type of training focuses on helping the learners to build conceptual models of the relevant areas, which entails developing acute problem-solving skills and relevant cognitive attitudes to inform behaviour.

There are four distinct differences between our approach and those of many other socialisation interventions:

1.   The focus is on developing interaction skills as a foundation for any other improvements in verbal, nonverbal and emotional behaviours.

2.   The intervention is developmentally geared to the adolescents' stage of cognitive development.

3.   The methodology is stretched across the line connecting current research on autistic spectrum disorders with what might conveniently be termed the applied philosophy of language.

4.   Roughly 25 per cent of the intervention modules are explicitly parent focused with contact time set aside for outside intervention hours.

Group screening issues

It is difficult to legislate for group size, but time is limited so one must establish a group size that will allow:

- reasonable levels of individual attention

- multiple opportunities for interactions

- completion of the session content

- manageability in terms of behaviour

- feedback opportunities.

Ideally, group participants will be matched for language skills and IQ. This point is worth repeating. Working with unmatched groups may lead to incomplete or uneven coverage of content and interfere with role play and rehearsal time.

Consider the case where a group of ten AS adolescents has one or two members with moderate to low language comprehension and expressive skills. Assume that the other members take a minute each to respond to a question or initiate an interaction. The unmatched lower functioning members may take six minutes to respond. Effectively each of the latter is equivalent to five people in the group as measured by response time. The group of ten therefore functions as a group with at least 15 members.

The mathematics of participation is quite simple. If each session is two hours long, and allowing for a break of 15 minutes in the middle plus five minutes settling in time at the beginning, only 100 minutes remain. If the group has ten members, then each member can expect ten minutes of individual attention. Participants listen and watch each other beneficially, but the formula drives home the point that participants in smaller groups receive more attention. A manageable group size is between six and eight adolescents. Once the group has more than eight people, consider either extending the length of the sessions or forming two groups. Large groups provide greater opportunities for attention drift. In mitigation, one should allow for some attrition, as the group is likely to contract slightly in the first few weeks due to a variety of factors beyond the therapist's control. Depending on the circumstances, we recommend starting with a group of no less than eight matched adolescents. The gender balance will probably favour males.

If the intervention is delivered within a school and during school time, attrition will be less than an outside of school service. There are a number of reasons ranging from convenience through to the presence of a ready audience favouring a school setting. However, irrespective of the setting, some adolescents may not be ready for group inclusion due to overwhelming social anxiety, major depressive illness, intense self-preoccupation, severe attention deficit hyperactivity disorder (ADHD) or entrenched oppositional defiant disorder (ODD). Some teenagers may need medication and others may need individual sessions with a therapist to facilitate preparation for group interaction.

In the short term, adolescents who are continually verbally abusive or lack self-control are not suitable participants. Such behaviours are intimidating and obstruct group cohesion. Their inclusion in a group should be deferred pending the results of external therapy and possibly medication. Furthermore, adolescents manifesting acute anxiety, severe depression or extreme self-preoccupation may have great difficulty learning and responding to cues and prompts. The very presence of others can be overwhelming. Preparatory therapy may be required.

Adolescents with unmanaged ADHD may be interruptive (without being abusive) and, again, not react to appropriate cues and prompts, especially around turn taking. Depending on the severity of the ADHD presentation, the therapist must decide how best to continue the adolescent's participation in the intervention. This may require that parents review medication options with their psychiatrist. The co-occurrence of ADHD with autistic spectrum disorders is high, and consequently there is a need to develop management strategies for those affected (Fallgatter *et al.* 2005; Sergeant *et al.* 2003; Sturm, Fernell and Gillberg 2004; Yoshida and Uchiyama 2004).

Those with ADHD and AS are impulsive and will interrupt, talk and change seats in total ignorance of their impact on other group members. This can be wearying and a therapist may find herself drawn into spending disproportionate amounts of time correcting the behaviour. A better strategy is to operate a system of signals based on a rule similar to 'three strikes and you are out'. The affected person is signalled (using a finger or a piece of coloured card) each time he or she violates turn taking. Three signals earns a period time (ten minutes, say) outside of the group. For safety's sake the person will need to be accompanied if asked to leave the group for this period of time. If these management strategies are not effective, then some form of suspension may be required during which individual therapy can be applied.

It may seem self-evident but it is important to make sure that each adolescent knows that he or she has a diagnosis of Asperger syndrome. Some parents misguidedly believe that hiding the diagnosis from a child is in the child's best interest. During latency years this may be true, but in adolescence the rationale is less sustainable. It is impossible to conduct an intervention for AS adolescents if one of the participants has been encouraged in the false belief that they do not have Asperger syndrome. Many issues will arise that probe self-knowledge of the daily impact of AS, and the intervention would halt if these were set aside for fear the topics would challenge parental preferences for nondisclosure.

A final issue to ponder when assembling a group is what set of assessment instruments will be relied upon to give the most accurate participant profiles. We have tended to rely on tests that require third-party (parent or guardian) input to get a picture of the communication and social disorders present in a participant. The following were found to be particularly helpful: the Children's Communication Checklist (revised version); the Vineland for adolescents and the Strengths and Difficulties Questionnaire (Bishop 1998; Sparrow, Balla and Cicchetti 1984). Participants will have an IQ score derived from the WISC before attending a group (Weschler 1992). They will also have completed the Strengths and Difficulties Questionnaire (Goodman 1999).

Pre- and post-testing

Screening of participants is recommended. Pre-intervention testing gives a measure of a participant's performance in several areas relating to self-regulation, self-sufficiency skills and social interaction abilities. The range of testing instruments available is extensive. However, the instruments listed below are established tests suitable for pre-intervention screening. The Vineland is suitable for pre- and post-intervention usage depending on the passage of time. If the time between the beginning and end of the intervention is not developmentally significant, the Vineland may be less suitable.

Tests of pragmatic language and language competence exist in various forms. Their applicability to AS studies is a moot point. Perhaps the most well-known are the Test of Language Competence and the Test of Pragmatic Language, (Phelps-Teraski and Phelps-Gunn 1992; Wiig and Secord 1989). Cultural bias, idiomatic fashions and language evolution challenge any attempt to develop broad but deeply insightful pragmatic assessment instruments. The dearth of such instruments for Asperger syndrome adolescents is striking, (Landa 2000).

There are arguably no standardised instruments to measure the full range of pragmatic capacities and discourse skills. Post-intervention testing is therefore problematical. The most reasonable course of action is to solicit regular feedback from parents and teachers about participants' interactions with peers. Third-party reports are not substitutes for a standardised test, but they are nevertheless essential markers of progress. They can be augmented by regular completion of short questionnaires about peer interaction frequencies such as the example in Appendix 7.

Vineland Scale

The Vineland Adaptive Behaviour Scales form part of an assessment gold standard. It has three versions, but the expanded form is most suited to autistic spectrum disorders (Sparrow *et al.* 1984). The expanded form can act as input to an individual education plan (IEP). It is geared towards measuring adaptive behaviour across four domains of daily life. These are Communication, Daily Living Skills, Socialisation and Motor Skills. In general people with autism score low in the Communication and Socialisation domains. The Vineland begins with the child's development as its reference point. Using a semi-structured interview with a parent it is possible to ascertain the skills which the child should have given his or her intellectual ability.

The Vineland consistently scores the Socialisation domain lowest for those with AS, though they perform better on Communication. Moreover, the distance between IQ scores and Vineland scores are very marked (Klin *et al.* 2000). This tends to reinforce research and clinical observations that people with AS with occasionally striking cognitive strengths are unable to turn these strengths to their advantage in the social domain.

Children's Communication Checklist

The Children's Communication Checklist (CCC) was devised by Dorothy Bishop to elicit measures of language impairment in children. Currently there are two versions of the CCC; the early version focuses on children between the ages of seven and nine (Bishop 1998). It is primarily designed for completion by teachers. In the latest version, the CCC has been expanded to include adolescents (Bishop 2003). This version is designed for completion by parents rather than teachers.

The CCC focuses on peculiarities in the content and use of language. Though a child's use of syntax and phonology may be relatively intact, their use of language is the locus of their specific language impairment (SLI). Early attempts to categorise SLI have proved difficult and controversial. Unlike instruments used in a formal test environment, Bishop's CCC is a rater based tool. The choice is justified on several grounds. First, the rater (teacher or parent) will have more complete appreciation of a child's behavioural range than can be encapsulated in a formal test environment. The rater will be aware of 'typical behaviour'. Second, certain behaviours may be difficult to elicit and measure in the test environment due to their infrequency. Introducing rater reports overcomes this difficulty.

The CCC rates features of language impairment that are considered clinically significant in reports but not readily amenable to measurement using conventional forms of assessment. CCC is a valuable assessment tool. If using the teacher version, teachers should know the child for at least three months. Due to limitations of the original version, including the possibility of rater bias and problems with cross-validation, use of the 2003 revised version with parents is preferable.

Strengths and Difficulties Questionnaire (SDQ)

The SDQ is a questionnaire about the behaviour of children from 3 to 16 years old. There are two versions: one for the child (from age 11) and one for the parent (and the teacher). The questions in both versions of the questionnaire address the same problems and behaviour, but the wording is different. An extended version includes an impact supplement that asks the respondent about whether the child or adolescent has a problem and what degree of distress, impairment and burden is associated with it (Goodman 1999; SDQINFO 2005).

The questionnaire consists of 25 questions divided over five areas: emotional symptoms, conduct problems, hyperactivity and inattention, peer relationship problems and prosocial behaviour. In our work, we found that the only area that adolescents and parents score equivalently is on peer relationship problems. In other areas, the adolescents minimise their difficulties relative to parental scores. The SDQ is not established as a post-intervention instrument, so improved scores in peer relationships post intervention must be judged cautiously.

Interaction modelling themes

The communication and social interaction themes elaborated in this intervention were derived from three sources:

- a literature review of extant literature and practices
- a survey of clinical specialists that had attempted social skills teaching with AS children in the past
- a survey of mundane social activities and potential challenges among typical and AS adolescents.

The box lists the top 20 themes that emerged. Additional themes include basic conversation initate–attend–listen–respond strategies and bullying. The former process is woven into all sessions. Bullying is such a universal problem in Asperger syndrome that it should be referenced in at least one session. However, this is not a substitute for schools implementing effective anti-bullying policies.

Social interaction themes

1. Asking for help – initiating

2. Asking for help – responding

3. Negotiation and compromise

4. Responding to an unfamiliar peer's request

5. Initiating with peers

6. Initiation and topic maintenance with familiar peers

7. Assessment of peer intentions

8. Accepting and responding to criticism

9. Coping with bullying – being assertive and seeking help

10. Self-monitoring and frustration control

11. Maintaining conversational focus in a formal setting

12. Avoiding giving offence

13. Probing for intentions in strangers

14. Accepting desires are not always satisfiable

15. Setting boundaries and assessing risk

16. Conversation: seeking positive attention

17. Managing anger when expectations not met

18. Recognising distress in others: empathy

19. Respecting social boundaries

20. Commonsense and impulse control

Themes can be addressed in several ways. Here is one suggestion, which is thorough if the intervention is run over a long period. First, ask each participant to put forward 'good' and 'bad' examples of the theme in action and in context: for example, a 'bad' way to ask for help in school would generally involve shouting at someone. Second, ask participants to explain to each other (in pairs) why one way is better than another. Third, model a role play that shows the wrong interaction style and ask the group to critique it. Next, guide the role play using the group feedback towards the right interaction style. All group participants get an opportunity to role play. Finally, within the group explore why the right way is the right way in terms of peer expectations. If the intervention is run as weekly sessions, this suggestion will need adaptation (see Chapter 8 for further advice).

Encourage active listening

Much has been written on active listening and it is almost impossible to conceive of an intervention that does not emphasise its importance. This is a recurrent theme and practised throughout the whole intervention. Essentially active listening is purposeful listening. The development of active listening skills requires that all listening be treated as a potential learning experience requiring attention on what is said and indicated by others. It discourages rushed judgements and 'snap' reactions to others. Active listening skills help those with AS to recognise cues for turn taking and not interrupting. Cutting off someone else's conversational turn is extremely irritating and people with AS require huge amounts of practice at developing and recognising appropriate cues and turn-taking strategies. The benefits of engaging in active listening are:

- minimisation of distractions
- focus is on present activity and interaction
- curbs interruptive tendency
- increased focus on topic relevance
- discouragement of daydreaming
- helps to ground friendships
- aids acceptance of criticism.

Again, it is important that a therapist regularly signals to parents that these strategies must be implemented and practised at home. Parents may be so habituated to their adolescent's dominant interaction style in the family that they fail to grasp its consequences for their adolescent outside the family setting. *Active listening must be practised at home by parents and their adolescents.*

Wherever possible use verbs not adjectives

The therapist should focus on using action words (or interaction words) rather than words that describe states. Rather than ask the group to describe how someone is feeling or the state he or she is in, ask him or her to produce the behaviour that is occurring. This is designed to help the group think in terms of social processes as ever-present events that peers navigate constantly. Verbs add concreteness to descriptions that adjectives lack. In dealing with the AS mindset this is important: for example, *The scared boy is running out of the classroom* is different from *The boy is running out of the classroom.* How can we tell he is scared? What is the behaviour that allows us to attribute the adjective? Perhaps he was flicking his eyes around, swivelling his head quickly, breathing heavily or crying tears. In any event, he was doing something that allowed us to conclude he was scared.

Not all verbs are action verbs. Verbs that describe mental activity are a case in point: believe, know, want, and so forth. These verbs describe states of mind that have to be inferred from interaction between behaviour and discourse. Careful observation and exploration of behaviour in communication is necessary.

Role play

Role plays are common to many therapies. Modelling solutions and strategies for interpersonal problem solving is a constant theme. There are debates in the literature, which need not concern us, about distinctions between drama, enactment and role play.

Role play influenced by psychodrama is often used to help children express angry, fearful or negative feelings. The children act out specific feelings through adopting particular roles (Stephenson 1993). In this mode, role play is less about finding strategies of interpersonal communication and more about the release or supervision of psychic strains experienced by the child. Helping children come to terms with loss is one example (Smith and Pennells 1993).

In our own work we have stayed away from dramatic role play because the dynamic in drama is one of conflict and catharsis, which may be emotionally confusing and overpowering for people with AS. Referring back to Chapter 2, the limbic system theory of autism explicitly hypothesises a deficient emotion-processing mechanism. Focusing on emotional development prior to enhancing a range of discourse interaction skills (largely cognitive processing tasks) may be a case of putting the cart before the horse. It is a debatable point, but we focus primarily on turning implicitly learnt abilities of the typical peer into explicitly realisable cognitive processes for the AS peer. However, almost any therapeutic approach or activity that facilitates people with AS engaging in social interaction is worthwhile.

Role play as a form of enactment of solutions by participants (without requiring anyone to adopt dramatic roles) is essential to aid the absorption and practice of the relevant capacities and skills. People with AS need to explore other people's points of view and role play is necessary. However, roles should be natural roles – peer roles – to assist the carryover into the environment of the AS adolescent. If roles are removed from that environment (e.g. an astronaut) the transfer will be minimal to nonexistent.

Role taking by the participants should only proceed once the theme and associated interaction difficulty have been explored. The problem scenario should be analysed along the lines of the conclusions in Chapter 3. As a rule of thumb, role plays should best begin from perspectives near to the perspective of the participants. Moving them away from these perspectives (rotating them through the perspectives of others) is a gradual process (Dowrick 1986). Some participants will progress more rapidly than others. Once the group is attuned to interaction with each other then role reversal is conceivable. Here a participant swaps a role with another. Again, it is stressed that roles should be naturalistic and relate to peers in the everyday environment.

Despite the apparent self-evident need for role play, it is not beyond criticism. Perhaps the most established concern is that the 'actors' will perform to fit the bias of the therapist rather than express themselves honestly. A second common criticism is that effective role plays may not carry over to the outside world. The 'stage' of the intervention may give a misleading impression of actual social interaction abilities. No doubt both of these criticisms have a certain validity. The only response is to examine the experiences of participants in the real world. At the end of the day, the group matters more than the method. Almost any therapy that facilitates people with AS engaging in social interaction is worthwhile.

Conversation

Conversation has been covered extensively in Chapter 3. What we wish to add here are a few tips on directing it in the group. First, conversation should be discussed with the participants. Learning what they understand by conversation will help tailor response to suit individual participants' needs. Most people with AS understand conversation as a type of input–output process. Information is provided or information is sought. However, the levels of depression and isolation experienced by AS adolescents indicate that these young people know that there is more to conversation than just information exchange.

Second, it is worthwhile listening to positive and negative conversational experiences they have had with peers. This will help the therapist understand the school and peer environment. Often, these adolescents have no idea why peers display such hostility towards them. They need assistance to unpick any assumptions about peers that are negative.

Third, the therapist should use short sentences initially until the group is relaxed. The main mechanism for facilitating conversation is to have each participant talk to his neighbour, then reverse roles and be an audience for his neighbour. Anxiety about 'failing in conversation' will be high, so a lot of encouragement is required. Topics should relate directly to the social interaction theme of the session. Topics should also relate to the school–home environment of the adolescents (even if one or two are not in school). Doubtless the participants will have their own expectations of sessions and it is important to factor these into the conversational practice.

Fourth, only constructive positive comments are allowed in conversation. This applies to the parents as much as to the adolescents. The exhortation to comment constructively cannot be repeated too often to families coping with autistic spectrum disorders. We deliberately go over this point again, as it is so important that it be emphasised repeatedly in the intervention.

Homework

The very term 'homework' conjures up drudgery and competition. For some in the group it has associations with years of academic underperformance and humiliation. If possible, avoid the term and use 'rehearsal work' or 'session refreshers'. School-attending adolescents are familiar with written homework and will probably complete it diligently. The question is whether written homework has a purpose.

Initially, it may help to add familiar structure to a session, but material on paper is not conversation, it is not interaction. The real homework begins outside the intervention when they attempt to practise what has been learnt in the intervention. As confidence within the group grows, encourage the adolescents to keep a tally of successful peer interactions. Apart from setting them a goal, it also provides informal feedback on their uptake of the pragmatic strategies and discourse skills.

Intervention outcomes

Rather than recapitulating on the points made above, this section tries to answer the question: what will be different? The first major result that should occur is the development of a cohesive 'social group'. If the intervention has effected a change, the adolescents will converse freely with one another, observe turn taking, exhibit appropriate social use of language and, most importantly, have some contact with one another outside the group setting. This can be accomplished using a phone with parental knowledge and consent. They will actually enjoy the experience of social interaction with peers in the group. To date those parents that have stayed the course (80%) have given overwhelmingly positive feedback about the intervention. They have consistently reported that their teenagers are:

- calmer, happier and more goal focused

- better adjusted in school according to teacher reports to parents

- making more overtures to peers

- experiencing more success in peer company.

Doreen was the mother a 16-year-old boy with AS named Fred. His IQ was in the average range but he had difficulty expressing himself in written form. His self-organisation skills were below those expected for his age. She said herself in a letter that if Fred was left at home he might 'pull down the television' while changing channels. He often left his homework 'in a mess'. In school Fred was perceived as aloof and morose by both teachers and classmates. He had been learning to play the drums on his own, even though the school encouraged teenage bands. After three months in the intervention, his mother reported that he had decided to overcome his anxiety and joined one of the bands that needed a drummer. She was convinced that Fred gained sufficient confidence and positive acclamation from his peers in the intervention to 'pluck up the courage' to reach out to his school peers. Crucial to this was the variety of strategies practised and examined in role play. Fred took a big step forward. It did not, however, settle all of his interaction difficulties but it did mean that he was no longer isolated in school and now had at least one foundation group of receptive peers.

Second, parents will have amended their communication style to reflect the principles of the programme. They will facilitate external social interactions among the group. Through harmonious operation of their support group the parents also function as positive role models for social interaction.

Trina was the single mother of Darren, a 16-year-old boy with AS. In Trina's own words 'Darren had a difficult time in school' and would leave for periods of weeks at a time due to anxiety and stress. Once Trina asked if we had covered 'anything on conversation' in the previous session. In fact, we had covered active listening. She reported that Darren had 'caught' her not listening to him as 'he went off into one of his rants' several times over the subsequent days. Usually, she would pick up a newspaper and read while he 'sounded off'. The newspaper was something of a sound barrier. However, she was stunned when he reprimanded her on several occasions and asked if she 'was enjoying the conversation'. Trina revisited a handout on pragmatics and realised that her own communication style with Darren was not modelling the desired listening and turn-taking strategies. Subsequently both mother and son made a pact to practise active listening strategies more frequently.

Third, reports of generalisation or carry over of learning within peer settings from parents and/or teachers should filter back. Many parents of AS adolescents regularly communicate with school. Improvements in the school setting may include teacher reports of improved self-confidence, greater ease in peer relations and increased participation in peer activities. It is important to issue the social interaction checklist on a regular basis to parents to ensure that important details of social activities are not missed.

Anita's son Jim was 15 years old with AS and an above average IQ. He was very satisfied with his academic studies. Also, he was fortunate in attending a school with well-defined policies for protecting marginalised children from bullying. Jim had been through half-a-dozen social skills courses and spent four years in drama classes without any improvement in peer relations. In school he kept to himself and regarded his classmates as 'dorks'. Over the years, teachers reported to his mother that while he seemed well adjusted in school, he was never observed in conversation with other peers beyond perfunctory exchanges. Anita recounted that Jim had no interest in 'hanging around' with peers where they lived. 'In the past, they would call to the door or call out to him to join them if we pulled up in the car, but he would shout f**k off at them over his shoulder and retreat into the house,' she recalled. Jim was not obviously depressed or unhappy but he was extremely anxious socially. Over a period of ten weeks in the intervention, Jim changed from wanting to run out the door at the end of a session, to demanding more break time so he could 'talk more with the others'. One evening when a session ran over time, parents came to the room to collect their sons and daughters. The group were chatting and being slightly boisterous. Anita appeared in the door and remarked, 'God, they're just like normal teenagers.' Subsequently, Jim went on a day trip with his class, the first ever. Anita was late picking him up from the school and with some trepidation sought him out. She was surprised to find him sitting on a wall with a group from his class and obviously comfortable with them. Since that time Jim has been on two other day trips and while he still does not have a firm friend (or does not want one perhaps) he now has more company and both his mother and his psychiatrist are impressed with his development.

Finally, while the focus is on improving capacities and skills in the participants, and the development of better interaction strategies, the intervention may not have the same positive effects equally across the group. It will happen that some participants will benefit more than others. This is why we emphasise *doing the most for the most*. The aspirations of the therapist may be high, which is the right attitude, but the social interaction goals of the intervention are modest: but a modest improvement in someone with AS may amount to a major improvement over time.

5 Video Modelling and Script Models

We devote this chapter to assessing the merits of using video modelling in an interaction skills intervention. We also touch upon the task of making one's own video resources. Our interest in video material is as an aid to cognitive restructuring. Video materials are used to challenge AS assumptions about the world. Appropriate material can also provide a glimpse of what is possible in the future with change. They provide visual materials which model and support explorations of role plays of situations that require adaptive behaviours, that is, appropriate social interaction capacities. It is for these reasons that video material should be sought out.

We emphasise at the outset that all materials must be available for viewing by parents upon request. A screening of sample video content should be organised for parents prior to seeking their consent. This gives them an opportunity to raise concerns and clarify any misconceptions. It also provides the therapist with an opportunity to explain the role of the video material clearly. In what follows, we use video modelling to refer primarily to pre-recorded clips of social situations – packaged solutions. This differs from the use of video modelling to record group and individual performance on tasks. In the latter, the video recording is used to give positive feedback with a view to strengthening individual or group efforts to master social techniques (Dowrick 1999; Kemenoff *et al.* 1995). There is little doubt that this is valuable but it requires:

- consent of the group and probably parents

- technical expertise in video production

- substantial commitment to edit raw footage to provide a positive self-image to the participant(s).

Historically, audiovisual material (video in our terms) was limited to playback through a conventional television. The development of multimedia computers, multimedia mobile phones, the internet and personal handheld computers presents a wide range of devices for playback of video. It is possible to adopt an anytime anywhere approach to using video within an intervention. In other words, few technological obstacles exist that would prevent the flexible use of video. However, one should not allow technological diversity to dictate the tailoring of the intervention. When the fundamental focus is on what is best for the adolescent within a group setting, using technology to shore up group work is a welcome but secondary bonus.

Granting that the technology for video delivery is accessible to most mental health services and schools and homes, the next question is what content is appropriate. This masks several dilemmas relating to content provisions for therapists, adolescents and even parents. Each group may require the same core content, but with different satellite modules depending on home usage or not. On the other hand, each group may require radically different content depending on the abilities of the group and the available therapeutic resources. The intervention in this book outlines core content because logically the latter option is impractical. Without common content across settings, it will be difficult to maintain consistency in delivery, focus and theme. Supplementary matters include whether the content should be specifically AS focused. Should clips of easily available material from peer television series and movies be preferred? There are no easy answers to these questions. Different institutional policies, availability of resources, plus therapeutic preferences will usually dictate practices.

Why bother with video?

Due to the ubiquity of television and cinema, almost everyone is an implicit expert on video production standards. Even if someone cannot offer a detailed critique of where a video is wrong, she or he will certainly discriminate between 'good' and 'bad' media content. Holding the viewer's attention was once the concern of drama, but increasingly other programme types compete aggressively for attention. Much of this competition is displayed to the styles of the various programmes, and in turn these have influenced the development of current affairs, science and documentary production standards (Hampe 1997). For example, a plethora of news channels is devoted to a production model based on novel means for situating the playing of media clips with interpretive voiceovers. Modern societies rely on visual representations of the world to convey information more than was possible in previous centuries. Unlike radio, the visual mode of representation dominates and has primacy.

In the social world, our interactions are also visually related one to another. Phone conversation is one small aspect of interaction that removes the visual cues but it is subsidiary to face-to-face communication. Effective social interaction requires embodied interaction with other people, and in turn this draws upon attention and observation skills. People with AS find remote interaction, through email and phone, easier than embodied interaction. Embodied interaction requires immersion in a social world with many different stimuli hurtling about, and that can be very confusing. The use of video materials in teaching social interaction skills is a safe compromise between remote interaction and full immersion. On the one hand, video can represent behaviour concisely, and on the other it allows the viewer to comment upon and explore mimicking the behaviour without negative outcomes. Video can be used to:

- stimulate discussion about difficult social situations

- represent packaged solutions to social problems

- aid cognitive restructuring through playback of participant performance

- explore consequences of interactions

- evaluate progress in recognising social cues

- improve recognition of facial expressions.

The power of video as an attention 'stimulant' is important in AS interventions. Not only does it help hold someone's attention, but it also draws the group into observing the behaviour of others and through that into exploring the perspectives of others. It allows repetitive analysis of particularly tricky situations for the adolescent. A human enacted role play can only be performed so many times with enthusiasm, but a video clip can be replayed many times without the same physical overhead.

In theory, video production allows free rein to create a range of scenarios and possible outcomes with developmentally matched peers, but in practice resources constrain the final production standards. Many therapists are more than capable of producing (or overseeing the production of) usable video material for an intervention by following guidelines (Long and Schenk 2002).

The downside to video usage is that if it is applied too extensively an intervention runs the risk of becoming too passive. A group will come to see the sessions as more like a trip to the cinema than an activity helping them towards social interaction. A second problem is access to appropriate materials. The amount of time required for an AS intervention to be deemed successful, and consequently the amount of material required, is unclear. Many experts indicate that near lifelong intervention support will be required for a percentage of people with AS (Attwood 1998; Howlin 1998, 2003; Howlin *et al.* 2004; Ozonoff *et al.* 2002). Hence, any commitment to producing video content has to be carefully balanced against cost, production knowledge and the inevitable time commitment. For instance, it is unlikely that a mainstream video production company would be in a position to make the most use of a set of scripts without the entire production being overseen by someone with expertise in AS. The risk is that the production company will use an established industry formula for producing instructional materials, ignoring the specific need to address deficits in the autistic mindset. In other words, the material should be feature specific to maximise its utility in an AS intervention.

A caveat about expectations

One of the initial aims of the intervention was to provide material for parents and adolescents for home use. The video materials addressed that need. The other objective was to tie the home use of material into access to an intervention programme. Again, for those who could access the programme, their resolve was strengthened. Over time it became clear that parents frequently had 'enough on their plates', and acting as home persuaders and tutors were demanding roles that not all could fulfil despite their commitment and determination.

In our own experience, and we stress this is our judgement rather than a standardised scientific result, video materials may create unrealistic expectations, especially in parents. Three observations on small-scale trials deserve comment. First, parental ability to 'talk through' the material with their adolescents was uneven. Varieties of reasons explain this gap. These range from educational attainment, parental motivation, adolescent willingness to collaborate with parents, and general problems with organising and structuring the activity. Second, parents were briefed on lesson plans and the type of commentary that accompanied each theme, but still the concepts and processes were very far removed from their backgrounds and everyday lives. Their own motivation to 'stick with' the videos was shaken. Finally, varying expectations of the video's capacity to effect change were noticeable. A small percentage of parents assumed that the videos would have an immediate corrective effect akin to taking a pill for a headache. Others were unsure if their enthusiasm for the materials was provoking exaggerated negative (or positive) reactions in the adolescents. Another set wanted to focus solely on specific themes that were problematical for their adolescents, but ignore other themes.

Once the prototyping experiment was complete, it was decided to continue with the video materials in a therapeutic setting and pursue a cut-down version with those parents who would undergo intensive training. Even then, adolescents are not keen to sit down with parents for instruction in social skills training. This is another reason why we emphasise the need for therapists to develop realistic expectations of what parents can do at home with the intervention. In some cases, getting an adolescent to attend even one session is a near miracle.

On a more scientific note, the learnability of facial expressions and emotions from video is a moot issue. A number of studies of facial expression recognition in AS have produced uneven results (Baron-Cohen *et al.* 2001; Barton *et al.* 2004; Celani, Battacchi and Arcidiacono 1999; Klin *et al.* 1999; Schultz *et al.* 2000). In the case of video, there is emerging research that people with AS may miss important social cues due to a tendency to focus on mouth rather than eyes (Klin *et al.* 2004). This latter result is important. Therapists should not assume that what they see in the eyes of the actors is also being seen by their group. It will be necessary to draw explicit attention to eye gaze details if participants are failing to pick them out with reasonable frequency.

Observational learning and video

Different sectors have used video modelling for many years to facilitate learning skills. The areas range over almost every field of human endeavour, from aircraft maintenance to woodturning. These videos are largely instructional by nature. They show the viewer how to tackle a specific task – learn a new skill. The world of commerce and management also uses video material to meet training needs, such as learning to use a computerised lending system or effectively interviewing an applicant for a job. Educating people to perform healthcare checks is another recent development. In principle, all instructional materials are trying to model the future for the person using the materials. The future shows a problem solved, a fresh skill learnt, and the mastery of new knowledge. Essential to the efficacy of these instructional videos is their reliance on the observational learning capacity of the viewer. If humans did not learn by observation, with instructional elaboration on key points, the production of such materials would be pointless.

In therapeutic settings, video materials are often admixtures of both styles – a dramatic reconstruction of a problem scenario accompanied by instructions to the therapist (or the client). The objective is to assist a person to move from maladaptive behaviour to adaptive behaviour. The dramatic component is often called a vignette or a scenario. It captures a slice of the world, usually a problem situation, which is reconstructed by actors. The reconstruction models the human dynamics involving speech, behaviour and emotions. These resources are also available on DVD with web support, increasing their flexibility and, at least in theory, providing rapid feedback to the end user on problems. Several instructional DVDs are available to therapists dealing with autistic spectrum disorders and any search of the internet will turn up new material on a regular basis. While resources exist for autistic children, there are few if any resources for Asperger syndrome adolescents (Nordin and Gillberg 1998). Even when video materials are available, how does one assess their value? There is certainly no theoretically pure answer to this question. The value of instructional video material is not simply locked up in the content. It entails the use of that content as well. The ability of a therapist to tailor the delivery and subsequent exploration to the expectations and needs of the group is a crucial factor in the process.

For our work, we have made 56 videos covering 23 communication themes. A range of individual professionals (the authors and two speech therapists) and two adolescent focus groups assessed the content of the video scripts before any production began. In terms of identifying and addressing deficits, the content has a sound educational base, is a rational expression of evidence-based clinical practice and expresses peer-appropriate behaviours, dress and speech – the latter marking the content as ecologically sound.

The videos were designed for a therapeutic role. There was a requirement that the main themes be addressable adequately in a short amount of time. For instance, if a theme required a 40-minute video, what time would be left for activities? The emphasis was therefore on short videos that focused more or less exclusively on one primary theme (obviously, a range of secondary themes is inherent in any social scenario). Predicted group variations in attention spans also influenced this choice.

The advantages of the videos in the intervention are largely due to the accessibility of themes. Accessibility saves time as the participants do not have to gear up for a role play without first seeing a visual guide. The therapist is therefore provided with more time to stimulate and manage interactions within the group. Second, pausing a video at key scenes enables discussion, modelling and enactment of consequences. For example, the therapist pauses at a scene during which an actor has been shouting his requests at another character. The group is asked to respond as the 'shouted at' character, producing a range of verbal, nonverbal and emotional comment. The video is then played and characters' responses are compared with group ones. Third, the videos provide the therapist with a ready collection of templates that can be called upon to illustrate details from a variety of perspectives. Finally, the reactions of participants to the videos often reveal idiosyncrasies not captured in any of the assessments. For example, one participant was completely unaware of the intent in an actor's tone of voice. In this case, whether a request was shouted or whispered was irrelevant to the adolescent. What mattered was that the request was logical and the other character either did or did not comply with it.

Script models: ineffective vs. effective

Almost every television series geared for adolescents has a dramatic structure which involves one adolescent doing the 'wrong thing', being found out and then after she or he has learnt the error of their behaviour, is provided with an opportunity for contrition and repair/restitution. Irrespective of whether a therapist is using purpose-designed content or clips from TV series and movies, if the fundamental social interaction difficulties are not identified within the group setting and opportunities provided to discuss (preferably view) appropriate social interactions, the material is irrelevant – no matter how rich the content.

The more content-rich the material, the greater the potential for distraction in an AS group. Weak Central Coherence (WCC) almost guarantees that there will be unevenness in the group when identifying relevant social details. However, if the material were required to reflect the peer social world, a content-starved offering would be ethically questionable and confound any generalisation attempts.

Tackling a range of adolescent maladaptive behaviours using a script model has a long tradition in various therapies. (Bledsoe, Smith and Simpson 2003; Bock 2001; Botvin 2000; Cook 2002; Dowrick 1986; Foxx *et al.* 1985; Gray 1994; Greenway 2000; Kazadin 1997; Ladd 1984; Myles 2001; Savidge *et al.* 2004; Webb *et al.* 2004; Whang, Fawcett and Mathews 1984; Whitehill *et al.* 1980). There is agreement that a social script is a recipe for following a social routine, with preconditions, planned steps and desired outcomes. The finer details vary, but without some grasp of social routines and their significance in social interaction it would be difficult to determine the motives of others. The typical person's capacity to internalise these routines and their applicability in specific circumstances is critical to directing his or her actions (Trillingsgaard 1999).

The social routines used by people with AS are often confused and lead to awkward moments – undesirable outcomes. Interaction routines producing outcomes that are unpleasant or isolate the person with AS, we deem ineffective social scripts. One common factor in the studies cited above is the principle that modelling adaptive behaviour, effective social scripts, is a necessary component in effecting change.

Script construction is strongly dependent upon the pragmatic capacities and categories discussed in Chapter 3. Generally, this is a repetitive process. A prototype script for a social interaction (SI) theme, including ineffective and effective versions, contains relevant pragmatic features and prosodic features. The prototype is assessed by a group of clinical experts and refined if necessary. The result is then brought to two separate adolescent focus groups – youth drama groups are ideal – and the language, idioms, behaviour and emotional content are assessed (Figure 5.1).

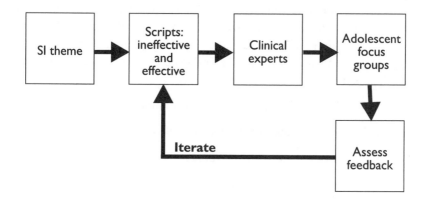

Figure 5.1 Script construction

If small refinements are needed, a revised script is assessed again by the clinicians. If radical refinements are required, the more inclusive process is repeated. During a video 'shoot', some small changes to scripts will probably be necessary to produce the required performance. Actors, even amateur actors, like to 'get into character'. Scripts should be fully elaborated before the production begins.

Arguably, there is no one effective social script model that will fit all adolescents with AS – unsurprising given that there is no biological marker of improvements in functioning over time. Our own working model for developing effective scripts involved the interaction themes mentioned earlier being presented ineffectively and effectively. Ineffective scripts contain pragmatic violations relevant to the theme. Effective scripts demonstrate appropriate pragmatic skills. Using compare-and-contrast strategies enables the adolescent to understand why certain interaction routines are ineffective and assists them to role play the features of effective interactions. A variety of pragmatic skills recurs in the scripts – greeting someone, acknowledging a question, and so forth. This reoccurrence reinforces their ubiquity and significance in peer interactions. The use of peer focus groups helped correct the narrative and language of the scripts. Appendix 6 provides a sample script illustrating ineffective and effective social interaction modes.

Video material is an aid to developing social judgements and interaction skills. It is critical to facilitate exploration and learning within the group that the social narrative, the interaction scaffolding, is unfolded slowly and logically. There is the risk that what is obvious to the therapist will be missed by the group, and occasionally what seems self-evident to group members may be overlooked by the therapist. In any AS group, there will be unevenness in comprehension. Some participants will notice one feature; others will notice something completely different and attach a contrary significance to it. The heterogeneity of AS makes it just so. The general considerations affecting the development and use of the videos included:

- no less than two and no more than four minutes length
- ineffective script presented prior to an effective script
- interaction difficulties discussed before solutions
- modelled solutions discussed and enacted
- peer relevance and consequences of 'bad' and 'good' interactions.

Solutions with effective social scripts should not appear 'out of the blue'. A certain amount of exploration within the group should hint at possible difficulties and the consequences of overcoming them. Once the modelled solution is shown, the central character should 'stand out' compared to his performance in the ineffective script. In any script, the core communication properties for exploration are the:

- verbal content
- nonverbal content
- emotional content of exchanges.

These properties are expressed in a social interaction routine consisting of the following:

1. Context (the setting influences interaction choices).

2. Purpose or goal identified (what is desired – perhaps several goals).

3. Preconditions for achieving the goal (what the character must know – the rules for the setting).

4. Required plan (what steps he must take to achieve his goal), the outcome(s) of his plan.

5. Consequences that follow for him and others.

Experimenting with the steps in a routine alters its efficacy. This process of experimentation (process of exploration) is shared with the group and is the lever for effecting change.

Example of video usage

A slightly edited sample script is shown in Appendix 6. It will be used to illustrate the role of video content. The first point to note is that the script, named 'The Library', has two versions. The first version exemplifies an ineffective social script. The second version is an effective social script. Each interaction theme has either two or three associated scripts, but only one version is deemed effective. Reiterating the point above, the purpose of each version is to assist the group explore a social scenario. The exploration includes discussion, enactment and problem-solving tasks.

Trite as it may sound, each script has a beginning, middle and end. The aim is to make the narrative and the 'lesson' of the script as explicit as possible. We do not suggest to the group that the central character has Asperger syndrome, but exploration of group experiences with AS is used to help understand the character's difficulties. This principle is followed to minimise biased responses from the group.

In the Library scenario, the adolescent seeks a particular book. The central theme of the video is *asking for help*. When the book is not in the expected place, he seeks the assistance of the library assistant. How is this introduced in the intervention? Three steps are required:

1. *Describe the initial task*: the therapist announces to the group that a video of a boy looking for a library book will be shown and the group will be asked some questions afterwards.

2. *Ensure group attention to content*: the video is shown and the therapist asks if the group understands it, but to 'make sure' the video is shown again.

3. *Explore and enact solutions*: the final step is the exploration of the social interactions that occurred. This will lead on to enacting solutions. This is the most important step.

If a participant professes not to understand an aspect of the video, other members of the group are invited to offer an explanation. The role of the therapist is to guide this process, keep it within time limits and steer it away from conflict and exhaustive qualification.

Before any further work, the group is asked to rate the boy on a social scale from one to ten, where one is 'terrible' and ten is 'brilliant' (Figure 5.2). Other video characters can be rated similarly. This is simply an exercise to get participants to focus on the characters. It is an important exercise as participants are also asked to justify the rating given to each character. In turn, this will reveal discrepancies between participants' grasp of salient features.

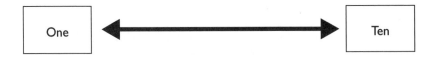

Figure 5.2 Rating a video character on a social scale from one to ten

Jim, for example, thought nothing of the boy shouting at the library assistant in the ineffective script. When asked why he reached this conclusion, he replied, 'Well, it is exactly what I would do myself. The assistant is there to assist, isn't she?' Tony on the other hand, did not notice any shouting in the scenario. His view was that the boy was a bit agitated, as he had been looking forward to studying the book that night. Myna, a girl, observed that library assistants were 'weird anyway' and she 'would not have a problem with anyone shouting at them'. Comments by others identified the shouting as an aggressive act.

One of the consistent results with this scenario is that less than a handful of the adolescents we have worked with have commented spontaneously on the tone used by the librarian. A typical therapist note for this scenario is as follows.

A teenager goes to the library to borrow a book. He checks the shelf but does not find it. He approaches the assistant to ask for assistance. The assistant is preoccupied sorting papers. In the first version, the teenager directly asks for the book without first getting her attention by making appropriate eye contact. He speaks in a raised voice and leans on her desk. He accepts her first hurried answer and leaves without clarifying when the book will be available again. He has no perspective on the assistant. He does not notice/ignores that she is busy.

In the second version, he waits until he gets her attention, adopts appropriate body language and engages in a clarifying dialogue. He has a perspective and pauses appropriately in between requests to obtain her attention. Eye contact, body language, speech and tone of voice are very important features to explore.

Teenager's goal(s):

- To borrow a particular book

Intervention goals:

- Learning to ask for help appropriately

Social goals:

- Asking for clarification
- Making a request
- Expressing gratitude/dissatisfaction
- Learning to cope with indifference/uncooperative responses

Subgoals:

- − Coping with rejection
- − Coping with rudeness

The group is asked to compare and contrast the ineffective script with the effective script along the lines above. Each participant should be given time to respond to questions. The group as a whole is allowed to discuss the features that were most noticeable to them and encouraged to suggest alternatives. These cognitive 'walk-through' exercises are essential preparation for any enactment of solutions.

The importance of purpose

It cannot be overstated that the exploration of any and every scenario is always conditioned by the autistic mindset. Exploring solutions or alternatives is pointless unless the purpose of the task is clearly understood and indeed justified to the group.

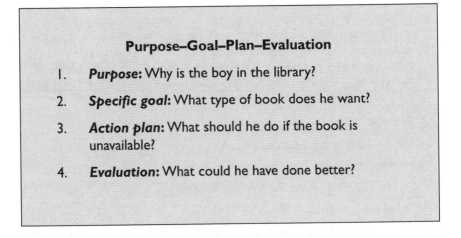

Purpose–Goal–Plan–Evaluation

1. *Purpose:* Why is the boy in the library?

2. *Specific goal:* What type of book does he want?

3. *Action plan:* What should he do if the book is unavailable?

4. *Evaluation:* What could he have done better?

Perspective on self and main character

Imitation and pretence relating to social problem solving are challenging for people with AS. In the box above, the focus is on the boy, his actions and intentions. To help explore the efficacy of his action plan, his social problem-solving skills, the participants are asked to help him by shifting perspective. To unseat passive following of the boy's behaviour the group is asked for a perspective on themselves and the central character.

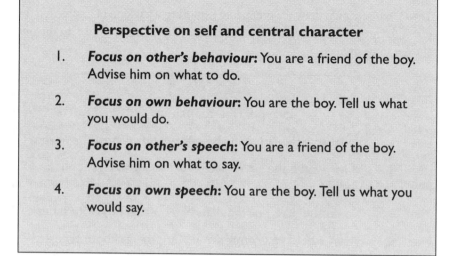

Perspective on self and central character

1. ***Focus on other's behaviour:*** You are a friend of the boy. Advise him on what to do.

2. ***Focus on own behaviour:*** You are the boy. Tell us what you would do.

3. ***Focus on other's speech:*** You are a friend of the boy. Advise him on what to say.

4. ***Focus on own speech:*** You are the boy. Tell us what you would say.

Research and clinical studies reveal that people with AS can appear quite competent problem solvers in the abstract (Klin, *et al.* 2000; Trillingsgaard 1999). However, once confronted with concrete situations, they behave very differently. In the 'real' social world, social interaction judgements and skills are required on demand. Exploring (2), and especially (3), are prequisites for any enactment of the scenario. It is extremely important in the case of (3) that participants say the actual words they would use. So rather than allowing someone to say: 'I would ask the girl to check again', the participant is required to speak his or her own words: 'Could you check that pile again please?'

In the scenario in question, the goal and plan are relatively easy to identify. After all, no small talk is required, no nuanced understanding of adolescent lingo intrudes and no social rejection is experienced. It is precisely because of these factors that such a scenario is a relatively comfortable one to explore at the beginning.

So far, the exploration with the group has focused on reacting to and understanding the world from the point of view of the boy, the central character. This is a prerequisite for enacting solutions and critiquing their effect, However, while necessary it is not sufficient in itself to complete the exploration of social interaction. Two other tasks must be completed.

Focus on perspective of other characters

The therapist should draw the group into exploring what kind of impression the girl is forming of the boy. A perspective-taking list of tasks similar to the one above can be applied.

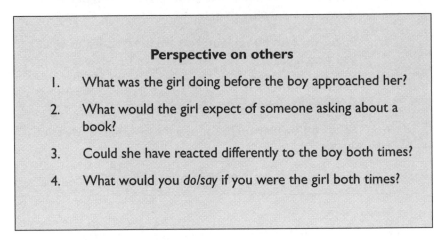

Perspective on others

1.   What was the girl doing before the boy approached her?

2.   What would the girl expect of someone asking about a book?

3.   Could she have reacted differently to the boy both times?

4.   What would you *do/say* if you were the girl both times?

The rationale for this set of tasks is part of dredging to the surface all that is implicit in the other person's expectations of interaction. Continual focus of the interaction expectations of other people cannot be overstated throughout the intervention. Before exploring task 4, the therapist may want to say something like this:

> The girl was busy before the boy approached her. She was preoccupied with her work. When people are very busy they expect other people to notice that they are busy. They tend not to notice other people who are not involved in their task. You need to get the attention of a busy person before he or she can communicate. The girl is doing a job and she expects people to enquire politely about books. Shouting and leaning on her desk, she interprets as rude behaviour. She could have decided not to answer the boy when he was rude, or even to call security to have him removed. When he was politely looking for her attention, she could have responded earlier. She gave the boy a very clear explanation about the book, however, and offered to hold it for him. She did that because she knows that library users expect reasonable explanations.

Consequences of behaviour on self and others

Any review of the vast swathe of (auto)biographical accounts of AS, reveals that almost everyone with AS has very little insight into the impact of their behaviour on others (Frith and Houston 2000; Gerland 1997; Grandin 1996; Holliday Willey 1999; Jackson 2002; Lawson 2003; Slater-Walker and Slater-Walker 2002). Irrespective of how one theorises about this absent ability, its acknowledgement in so many studies is a profound challenge to any intervention. Successful interaction is conditioned by the expectations of others. The consequences of AS behaviour require detailed exploration.

The strategies we favour draw upon the strengths of the AS mindset and encourage change as a means of mitigating other problems. In the first instance, clear logical explanations of behavioural impact are focused upon the conflict between the desired outcome and the actual outcome. Second, changing behaviour can bring rewards. If peers are annoying at times, reacting to them in a manner that provokes ridicule is a strategy designed to increase depression and isolation. Consequently, getting peers to react differently is founded on changes in the AS adolescent interaction styles. Change is dialogical. The interface between self and peers has to become more adaptive, but the leader in the process is the adolescent with AS (with school support one would hope). In other words, peers will not recognise that someone has adapted and changed their interaction style unless she or he shows that to be the case. Social interaction skills appropriate to context must be demonstrated.

It is useful to discuss with the group members their own experiences of how their behaviour got them into trouble or caused them pain and upset. Likewise they should be encouraged to report when their behaviour with peers brought them respect and satisfaction. This must be amplified as much as possible. Also, the AS adolescent by contrasting the ineffective with effective interaction styles is confronted with the rewards of the effective style. The main principles of cooperation and reciprocity to explore are as follows:

1. If you want to achieve a goal, behave in a way with others that will maximise your chances of succeeding.

2. Other people have memories. Offending someone today does not imply that he will have forgotten the event tomorrow just because you have.

3. Evolution and history teach us that cooperation is better in the longer term than non-cooperation.

4. Helping someone today makes it more likely that they will help you.

5. There is always tomorrow and that gives you a second chance, but not always.

The usefulness of the video material comes into play at one level very concretely helping enact a solution – and at another speculatively – exploring within the group a range of consequences from the undesirable to the desirable. This may be a long process.

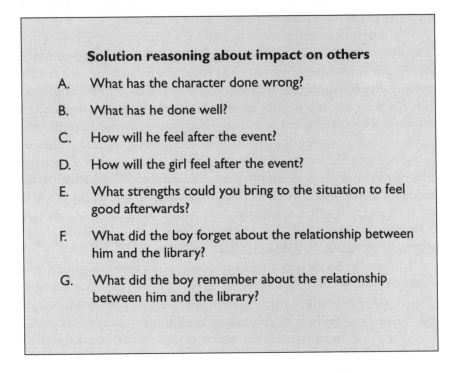

Solution reasoning about impact on others

A.   What has the character done wrong?

B.   What has he done well?

C.   How will he feel after the event?

D.   How will the girl feel after the event?

E.   What strengths could you bring to the situation to feel good afterwards?

F.   What did the boy forget about the relationship between him and the library?

G.   What did the boy remember about the relationship between him and the library?

One of the benefits in focusing on consequences is the opening up of space to consider the possibility of change. Video-modelled solutions show the benefits of changing from one mode of interaction to another more socially integrated mode. This feeds the AS mindset's need for *proof* that change is worthwhile. Many AS adolescents are reluctant to experiment with change in style. A key influence is the AS preference for routine, ritual and sameness. Hence, persuading someone with AS to tackle a task differently has to be linked to demonstrating *logically* the beneficial outcomes. With video, a therapist is not left simply to argue the case, but also has powerful visual aids to draw upon. We summarise the linkages below:

- Verbal discussion opens up the possibility of intellectual change.

- Video modelling illustrates the possibility concretely.

- Enactment helps learn and solidify the required interaction methods in the group.

- Reversing demoralisation allows the possibility of experimentation and practice in the world of peers.

No videos: what can I do?

The message of this section is blunt: everyone can make videos with appropriate team input. Video production is a collaborative process. Capturing raw footage requires a camera operator, probably someone to manage sound, a director, actors and a bundle of scripts. To produce a usable video, either access to expertise or a willingness to learn video editing skills is necessary. Everything on top of that is moving you towards professional video production.

Let us be clear, we are not talking about merely pointing a camera at a group of actors and packing the resulting footage away as a 'video'. At the very least an instructional video, even one with dramatic qualities, is:

- a sequence of visual images organised to tell a story

- a communication to an intended audience

- the result of careful editing of images to secure the narrative

- part craft and part science in therapeutic settings

- rarely as perfect as the one produced by your critics.

Many youth drama groups are more than willing to take on the dramatic tasks required. It may be possible to persuade the group to participate at a later stage – at least to allow them to critique their own social problem-solving skills during role plays. However, one should allow for group members opting out of video recording.

The content of videos comes from their scripts. Making a video requires judging if the balance between the visual and the audio is just right or too much in one direction. In the case of videos for an AS intervention, more explicit information is needed along both dimensions. Adequate acting performances can be obtained with a minimal understanding of directing (Weston 1996).

The primary quality of video, even instructional video of the sort we use, is that it is a visual medium. The emphasis during production has to be on the visual components capturing the story. If the narrative of a video is confusing to your audience, it is probably not worth using.

A video is not a radio play with visual images tagged on for enjoyment. The actual visual images have to tell their own narrative. Admittedly, certain activities lend themselves more easily to visual narrative. Contrast a video of someone building a bookcase with one dealing with marital therapy.

A video that is designed with instructional requirements in mind is not a piece of objective documentary work. It is a recreation of events for the camera. In the case of videos displaying various types of adolescent social interaction, these are also recreations of possible slices of the social experiences of adolescents. It is imperative therefore that they appear convincing. This requirement for *verisimilitude* entails that clothes, speech, posture and settings are consistent with contemporary adolescent life. While some level of compromise is allowable, it is best when it is minimal.

In the event that video material is completely unavailable irrespective of content, the group can still use role plays to enact social scenarios. Given the current state of technology and the huge variety of films and television series available on DVDs, it is unlikely in the extreme that material cannot be assembled over time from different sources that will be useful. Do not despair. The material is out there.

Conclusions

The primary role for video in an intervention is that of an exemplar. The material helps express both aurally and visually social interaction scenarios that require a range of social problem solving abilities and skills. Video materials are aids, means to ends, not an end in themselves.

Video material must be used in a highly disciplined manner, which is why we emphasise the importance of rehearsal. A common criticism of video content is that it encourages passive reaction rather than dynamic interaction. This is a risk if sessions become video bound rather than interaction focused. The pause and stop buttons should be used to provoke and stimulate reactions and interactions at crucial scenes.

To stimulate interest in the session topic and any role play to follow, it is prudent to play the video early in the session. Undoubtedly, there will be sessions where the introduction of video material is premature. In these situations, the key processes may require elaboration in a previous session. For example, *friendship* is not something that can be run through with ease, no matter how much or how little video material is on hand. Likewise, if a scenario is rich in verbal, nonverbal and emotion content, a gradual approach to identifying salient features will be more useful initially. Often the initial viewing will require utterance by utterance and gesture by gesture analysis. Hence, stepwise concentration on short scenes builds up to a complete analysis and elaboration of the scenario.

There is always a residual tension facing the therapist between the extents to which participants should be encouraged to model a specific solution and allowing them to be themselves. Since the intervention is designed to equip AS adolescents with successful strategies for social interaction, a commitment to changing the adolescents' mindset follows logically. Allowing the adolescents to be themselves in reaching for solutions may simply reinforce maladaptive strategies that have been unsuccessful in the past. The point is not that the group should be 'like' the socially efficacious video actors, but that the cohort of abilities displayed by the actors is peeled back. The vast majority of the adolescents coming to the intervention are there because their social world is not accommodating to them. The intervention seeks to improve their lot and alleviate their anxiety, depression and isolation. The principles, methods and objective espouse cognitive restructuring, which implies some level of change in the self. If modelling the video solutions is producing social success, this is a worthwhile outcome.

6 Format of the Sessions

In this chapter we describe the generic structure of a session and outline how a topic is elaborated with the AS adolescents and their parents. Sessions have a similar structure, whether adolescents or parents are involved. The structure should not be embraced as a straitjacket, but every session should clearly signal a structure to the participants:

1. Standard rules governing participation and behaviour:
   - Group recall of activities since last session.

2. Topic(s) for the current session:
   - Objectives for therapists
   - Delivery structure.

3. Activities and goals for the session:
   - Scenario for role play (presence varies from session to session)
   - Notes for the therapist (optional)
   - Speaking notes for use with adolescents (optional).

What to note?

Throughout the intervention, the group will evolve and the group dynamics will change. A careful record of activities is a useful source of information on the changes within the group and changing relationships between group participants and the therapist.

It is time consuming but necessary to make careful note of the verbal, non-verbal and emotional contributions of each participant. If permitted a video camera is useful, but a microphone and recorder is a less intrusive option. Conversational recording provides a useful measure of who is interacting, for how long and how successfully.

Frequencies and patterns of initiation and interaction among the group should be noted. Undoubtedly, an amount of unevenness will be noticed. The frequency of initiation refers to the number of times an individual volunteers an interaction with the therapist or members of the group. The pattern of initiation refers to regularities in the manner in which someone initiates. The categories in Chapter 3 are the basic identifiers.

Some participants will initiate interactions more frequently than others. Some may display such enthusiasm for initiation that they unintentionally smother the participation of others. On the other hand, others may be poor at initiating but will respond to an initiation from others. Reviewing notes from a previous session should prime a therapist to monitor these behaviours.

Initiation patterns may have a wide disparity of styles. Some participants will raise a hand to signal that they are ready to initiate with the therapist, and possibly other participants. Another set may simply speak out unprompted and interrupt others. Scrutinising initiation patterns will help tailor the intervention. Given the pronounced difficulties people with AS have with initiation, an accurate record of these patterns is invaluable.

If initiation is one side of the coin, turn taking is the other. Turn taking is intrinsic to *reciprocal communication*. In the beginning, anxiety and uneasiness in each other's company imposes a false turn taking. It is false in the sense that it does not spring from grasping pragmatic requirements and discourse skills. Instead, it arises from social anxiety and fear of failure. As the group evolves, this anxiety should disappear and adherence to turn taking becomes a problem. Noting the absence, presence and violation of turn taking will assist tailoring the intervention. Identifying pragmatically valid turn taking is sometimes difficult. It can be masked by randomness and interruptions.

Seamus was a 15-year-old boy with AS. He attended a private school where he excelled at homework. However, he had little interest in interacting with his peers and tended to keep his own company. Over time, in the intervention group setting, he became very relaxed and enjoyed meeting the other adolescents and conversing. Careful examination of his inputs indicated that despite superficially seeming to engage in conversation, he spent less than a third of his time actually following topics introduced by others. His conversation with others mostly consisted of comments and interjections with little regard for appropriate turn-taking rules or assessing the reaction of others to his inputs. Nevertheless, his behaviour was not unusual in the group at that stage and was not commented upon by any of his peers.

The paradox in Seamus's case is that he went from being uncommunicative in school to being inappropriately communicative in the group for large periods of time. In order to grasp and practise active listening and turn taking, Seamus required intense management within the group. Seamus's case is not unusual. In fact, as a group gels, more than one Seamus may be present.

Any revelations with implications for the mental or physical well-being of an adolescent should be noted and brought to the parents' attention as soon as possible. For instance, if an adolescent reports bullying or ridicule, depressive or suicidal thoughts, or exposure to any psychologically or physically harmful situations, informing the parents is mandatory.

Parent sessions

Parents of AS adolescents are often demoralised. Parents and adolescent are part of a family unit if not an entire unit themselves. Over many years they have been meeting the demands of having a child with AS. Many parents have been ground down by the impact of their child's social difficulties. Some parents have AS which may be placing additional pressure on marital relations. Now they face the challenge of a child growing into an adolescent and the new problems this entails. Parents will need a lot of encouragement and reminders about their crucial role in the development of their adolescent's opportunities for social interaction.

Parents are one of the pillars of this intervention. Depending on a therapist's expectations, parental capacities may at times seem to oscillate between strength and a weakness. However, as the relationship between therapist(s) and parents develops, a cooperative bridge will form. Parental attachment to the intervention is dependent upon the amount of support they receive from the sessions and from improvements in their adolescents' behaviours and social interactions. Their attachment is subordinate, however, to their adolescents' attachment to the intervention. This is conveyed to parents by the adolescent's willingness to return to the next session. Parents should have the therapist's expectations of them explained in simple language. From a therapist's perspective their roles are:

- to engage in active listening with the adolescent

- to practise positive comment as consistently as possible

- to assist with modelling targeted cognitions and behaviour

- to provide feedback on adolescent's behaviour through relevant questionnaires

- to collect observational data for analysis

- to provide increased peer interaction opportunities for adolescent.

When delivering parent-related sessions, one must grasp that parents are not receiving just a consultation but are active participants in the learning process. They have definite coaching and modelling roles. Where parents act as if they are onlookers to the process, the therapist has the task of diplomatically steering them back towards involvement in the activities. At the end of each session parents should be notified of the topic and asked to help their son or daughter practise the required skills.

A therapist may occasionally look upon a parent or adolescent as a reluctant participant – 'everything has to dragged out of them'. This demeanour may not signal reluctance but a discrepancy between the perspectives and expectations of both parties. Discrepancies can confuse judgements about what should be done with the reality of what can be done.

Let us face reality here also. Very few adolescents will be enamoured with the idea that their parents will coach them in social interactions, let alone model what is required. Be mindful that whatever compliance issues arise with the adolescents, parents may have to contend with additional hurdles due to work and family responsibilities. The bottom line is not to equate parental enthusiasm for the intervention with active daily pursuance of all the intervention objectives. It is simply not possible in all cases.

Adolescent sessions

All adolescent sessions should begin with a recapitulation of the rules, even if eventually the recapitulation becomes a ritual over time. The rules give predictable structure to the group environment as they lay out behavioural and interaction expectations.

Every session is directed towards group interactions and activities. If too much information is displayed on overheads or handouts, or the therapist gives long verbal explanations, the group will be deprived of interaction opportunities and attention will wane. As a role model, the therapist must demonstrate excellent active listening skills. This means focusing on the group, responding to their interactions, offering guidance, directing activities, acknowledging their inputs and displaying humour. All this is done with reference to developing pragmatic capacities and discourse skills.

The therapist should be enthusiastic about the participants' input, especially their performance in role plays. Make a point of bringing comments or suggestions by individuals to the attention of the whole group for acknowledgement. Use the adolescents' hobbies to help them initiate conversation with one another. Several of them will probably have overlapping hobbies (usually involving factual studies such as history or science). Computer video games are an almost ubiquitous passion. Where common interests arise, they are harnessed to ground conversational activities: 'Who has played game X in the past? Great! Tell the group a little about the characters'. A number of participants can be brought in on this topic.

In the initial sessions, revealing one's own hobbies (as an adolescent) will help the participants elaborate on their own hobbies. Lead them into conversation when necessary. Respect and take a probing interest in their hobbies, which are usually their passions.

In terms of equity, adolescent sessions should ensure that everyone gets a chance to participate equally. The emphasis is placed on producing conversation. Monosyllabic answers are not enough. Conversation must be steered along gradually but with a focus on the goals of each session.

Feedback to parents

The role of the therapist with parents is multifaceted. In dealing with parents, a therapist is expected to fulfil the following:

1. Use language that can 'reach' the parents. Any group of parents will have an uneven knowledge of AS. It is important that key objectives of the intervention be explained to parents in terms that (a) they understand and (b) relate to specific features of AS which they have observed.

2. Take them through a synopsis of the intervention and address their concerns about confidentiality and respecting their son or daughter's condition.

3. Explain the objectives behind the use of 'technical' phrases such as pragmatic language skills, social problem solving and so forth. These sessions encourage and equip parents to examine their own conversational styles and social negotiation skills. The objective is to assist parents revise their behaviours where the latter are reinforcing AS traits in the adolescents.

4. Emphasise that they have definite roles. The parents are required to organise 'real-world' social interaction contexts to facilitate and assess skill transference. The efficacy of the intervention is dependent upon skills transferring to the real world, i.e. the world of peers. Regular feedback from parents is necessary to evaluate the effectiveness of the intervention, or to modify its delivery.

5. Remind parents regularly about their role in the intervention and the ongoing importance of monitoring of communications skills within the family and school. Enquire about and congratulate parents on any changes they have made in their own communication patterns. Congratulate them on positive communication efforts.

It is helpful to give parents positive feedback about their child's progress in the group sessions. Parents may have specific issues that they would like addressed in the intervention. This is not always possible. The issues may be too specific for the setting. It should be explained to parents that their concerns have been noted and they will be assessed for inclusion in the intervention. Regular contact with parents is recommended after each session as an additional quality control measure.

Feedback to adolescents

Maintaining a positive constructive disposition towards the group will help them restructure their own cognitions. Everyone's input should be equally valued and the therapist should show the group that this is the case. Feedback that is encouraging and constructive builds confidence. When an activity or an interaction needs to be redone, it is preferable to comment, 'That was really a great effort. Can we try a slight variation on that now okay?' It is useful to remember that in their daily lives many of the participants receive little positive affirmation.

Feedback to the adolescents should be largely positive for efforts made and positive outcomes achieved. It should encourage participants to re-engineer an interaction strategy if necessary.

Humour and relaxation

Building trust and respect is essential to the viability of the group and the effectiveness of the intervention. A therapist must aid the group in learning to trust each other, which for most will be a novel peer experience compared with school. This means practising interaction activities, ensuring the expression of constructive comment, banning ridicule, and plenty of intelligent praise.

Relaxation is intrinsic to this process. Relaxed participants will be less anxious and more open to learning and interaction activities. Helpful exercises are in abundance. We adapted a variation that is well established in group therapy (Appendix 1). Humour is a powerful relaxant. The use of humour with AS adolescents is directed towards relaxation and anxiety management. One technique that the AS adolescents seem to enjoy is 'zany' self-deprecating humour. The purpose of off-beat humour is to tap the tangential orientation of the AS mindset. Think of it as akin to an 'I am on your wavelength' signal to the group.

Humour is so important in this form of therapy that we will dwell on it for a while longer. Several participants, almost certainly, will have a history of drifting from one social skills programme to another without experiencing an improvement in either their confidence or self-image. People with histories of 'failure' on other programmes, will not have high expectations of yet another intervention. Proving that the learning process can be enjoyable requires different strategies within the group and with different members of the group. These demands lean heavily upon a therapist's resourcefulness, that is, creative thinking and command of humour.

The aim of humour is not to tell the group 'I'm a funny person' or 'Wasn't that a great joke? Now like me better.' Humour signals that everyone is there to enjoy themselves. It also signals a light-hearted component to the sessions: we are going to have fun and learn! Frequently, mistakes will occur in a session, either with equipment or within one's delivery. A therapist should use these events to show the group how to respond to the unexpected flexibly. These occasions are used to develop humorous responses while exhibiting a capacity for developing alternatives. The therapist is also a fallible role model.

Rules for everyone

People with AS prefer structure and predictability. Inserting these components into the delivery of the intervention reduces anxiety and increases the likelihood of relaxation and openness to learning. It is essential that everyone, both therapists and participants, clearly understand and endorse the set of rules that will govern participation in the group. Once the rules are explicit, they can be invoked when a dispute or behaviour that is not conducive to positive social interaction occurs. The invocation of arbitrary rules to 'fix' a situation is among the worst 'crimes' from the perspective of the AS adolescents. The concrete, literal and logical mindset associated with AS always prefers explicit statements of rules. It is unwise to assume otherwise.

If the intervention is delivered in an institutional setting then rules governing the removal of participants from the group are probably in place. Otherwise, it is necessary to frame rules that allow the therapist to request the removal of a participant. Participants should have an opportunity to discuss and formally accept these rules before the intervention continues. Reasons for removing a participant vary from persistent non-participation through to aggression towards other group members. It is worth noting that occasionally participants can be traumatised by a group setting, though this may not be immediately evident in a large group. It may be unnoticeable to the therapist, but for some hypersensitive adolescents with AS even a faint imprint of a common social experience can evoke the recall of a past trauma. Affected participants, overpowered by their anxiety, may not return to the group.

In the opening sessions it is very important to focus on creating a safe place for the group. All the participants will gradually feel secure. It is essential to diminish their anxiety as the intervention progresses. The rules will help here. In certain cases, those with undiminished or even heightened anxiety will probably leave the group, despite the reassurance of the rules.

> All praise should have definite information content, with praise given for effort and any small step towards social interaction: e.g. *'That's an interesting/challenging/unusual point, I'll ask you to develop that later in a conversation with the person beside you.'* All interactions initiated by the therapist should be goal focused.

While there are many language issues to focus upon, an important one is the use of verbs rather than adjectives during group interactions. A common complaint from tutors of creative writing courses is the misuse of adjectives to describe a state when the scene requires verbs that describe action. The actions of others reveal their thoughts and intentions. This is an important point. Verbs belong to the action world, the world of human behaviour and interaction. Failure to comprehend nonverbal communication (actions or behaviours) is a key characteristic of AS. Hence, encouraging more use of verbs in the group is part of a restructuring process where they begin to perceive the world as a place of interaction between people. It is equally important to encourage the parents to use more verbs at home.

Introducing a topic

The therapist is a constant role model for the group. He or she demonstrates pragmatic capacities and discourse skills continuously to the group. Topics should be introduced with direct statements:

> This evening we will explore asking for help. We will talk about this as it might happen at school, at home or with other teenagers. So, I want each of you to tell the group about asking for help in those situations in the next 20 minutes and then we will do XYZ.

It is easier for the group if this is on an overhead as well:

- Identify what you want to talk about.

- Elaborate on it a little to give more context.

- Ask the other person(s) for his or her opinion.

- Listen to what they have to say.

- Signal a shift to the next topic.

- Close off the first topic (or conversation).

Towards the last third of the session, this structure of the pragmatic capacity and any associated discourse skill is explicitly revealed to the group and participants are asked to model it between themselves in role plays.

Other features can be dealt with similarly, such as topic maintenance, shifting, repairs, discourse skills. The strategy involves modelling the desired feature(s) while addressing a specific social interaction theme, and then re-analysing (*make explicit*) what has already been modelled (*shown*). Therefore, the group are practising specific social interaction strategies tied to themes, and practising the cross-contextual skills essential to effective social interaction.

Maintaining flow

The fundamental principle in the group setting is: *keep everything highly interactive*. Keep the participants alert and on their toes. Minimise the use of predictable styles of questioning. For example, if everyone is in a circle, move through the circle clockwise, anticlockwise, every second person, and so on. An element of the unpredictable will force the group members to pay closer attention. Keeping the group alert will make the sessions more exciting for everyone.

When group members interact with either the therapist or each other, enforce the use of first names. For example, in the early sessions during conversational practice, it is quite common for a participant to ask the therapist for the name of their conversation partner, '*I don't remember his name*'. Instruct the participant to ask his or her partner, '*What do you do when you want to know someone's name?*' This is a basic rule, but central to building basic social skills. To reinforce name learning, change the participants' seating preferences from session to session. This will prevent early exclusion of more anxious or vulnerable members and impede the development of a dominant clique. Likewise, if one participant is 'stuck' for conversation, select another participant to help him.

Try to give every person in the group equal participatory time – not always achievable. Enthusiastic members of the group will want to participate more frequently. Use their enthusiasm to help them master turn taking and interaction sequencing. Restrict interruptions for the same reasons.

Keep to the formula?

Issues of pressing importance to participants in the group may arise that will influence the session schedule. Among the instances that spring to mind is one in particular that involved betrayal of friendship and the theft of money. The adolescent affected was very troubled by the incident and one of his parents was very keen to have his reactions explored. Serendipitously, we have a number of scenarios that address 'false friends' and 'being conned'.

David was 14 years old and was diagnosed with AS at the age of 11 years. He had been on a school day trip with his classmates when another boy, new to the school, asked him for a loan of money to buy a sandwich and a soft drink. David gave him more than was required and asked the boy to purchase a similar snack for him. When the boy returned after 20 minutes, he had a portion of French fries, a sandwich roll and a large drink for himself. David asked for his meal. The boy apologised and told David he left it on the counter of the café with David's change from the money he lent. David was surprised and confused. The boy again explained how he had purchased David's meal but left it plus the surplus money on the counter. It was a misunderstanding. He assumed David was coming to collect his meal and change. For a week afterwards David became preoccupied with trying to rationalise the events. The boy had been friendly with him on the trip. Surely he could not have deliberately cheated him? His parents described his mood as swinging between being 'crushed' and 'murderous'. The school was informed about the event and managed to extract some degree of restitution from the other boy. David's confidence however was deeply shaken.

We decided not to raise David's experience directly but the general issue was raised in the group setting. He could then report his own experience if he wished. When the general issue was raised in the group, we discovered that everyone there had been 'conned' to one extent or the other. It was a very pertinent concern and we devoted additional sessions to exploring the mechanisms and effects of the behaviour. The rule of thumb we apply for extending a session or amending a schedule is whether the issue that has arisen is one of relevance to the majority of the group. If it is and there is the interest we amend the schedule.

Friendship in all its guises will always be a painful issue for adolescents with AS. The therapist should be prepared for a certain amount of group uneasiness around this topic. Handling the topic sensitively does not guarantee that individual participants will not feel pain. It is unfortunate when this occurs, but perhaps unavoidable unless the topic is avoided – not a sensible option.

Another potentially destabilising topic is sexuality, more accurately sexual relations. In our experience, we found few teenagers with AS sufficiently emotionally primed to grapple with the relevant issues meaningfully. For example, in one session we explore 'the disco' and the self-image of adolescents. Few AS adolescents we meet have ever been to a disco, and fewer still have danced with a member of the opposite sex. This may not be everyone's experience, but it is ours.

Adults with AS can react unpredictably to information about sexual relations. One therapist, in charge of a group, mentioned that after her first session one or two of the group asked when they would get their first kiss. In previous work we addressed issues of sexuality that are relevant for this age group, see (Harpur et al. 2003, ch. 7).

Checking homework

Since most of the group are likely to be in school, homework should be fun, not too challenging and avoid damaging existing school study schedules. All homework should focus on interacting with peers and peer interests. For example, ask the group to read the computer game, movie and music pages of a weekly newspaper. This is used to enhance common ground with peers. Paper-based homework has a role but a lesser role than speech-based homework.

Conclusions

Many issues confront the delivery of interventions to those with Asperger syndrome. The inclusion of parents in the equation adds a layer of complexity, but it is essential to involve parents for all the reasons outlined. A good working relationship with parents is necessary. Parental feedback from home and school is vital to determining the progress of individual participants.

Expectations vary across groups and within groups. As far as possible the therapist should acknowledge these expectations. Tailoring delivery of the intervention to address these expectations is important. Despite the very large body of scientific research into autism, very little has been done to account for motivational problems which afflict many on the spectrum. Depression and motivational torpor are likely to shadow any intervention for a period. Accurate recording of interactions, strengths and behaviours should be undertaken if resources permit.

Modelling takes place on two levels: direct modelling of strategies associated with a specific theme and indirect modelling of cross-context pragmatic capacities and discourse skills. Ultimately, everything the therapist does must 'touch base' with these features.

Adolescents enjoy constructive positive feedback. The intervention may be the one place they receive it.

7 Problems and Solution Tips

Increased rates of psychiatric problems in individuals and families coping with autism have been established in a number of studies (Nordin and Gillberg 1998; Piven *et al.* 1991; Sturm *et al.* 2004). It is likely that anyone on the autistic spectrum attending an intervention will manifest problems related to the condition that brought them into intervention in the first place. They may have problems in different areas of functioning, with varying levels of severity. The presence of psychiatric and emotional problems, or comorbidity, with Asperger syndrome has been reported in numerous studies, including Hans Asperger's original work. Several recent reviews of comorbidity have been published (Ghaziuddin 2005; Gillberg 2002). The majority of these conditions may be comorbid with AS due to underlying neurological factors. The reactions of family and peers impact greatly on the adolescent with Asperger syndrome. Depression and motivational torpor may arise due to the experiences of the person with AS in the world (not ruling out an underlying neurological sensitivity to these conditions, however). The over-representation of emotional disorders among this group has been noted in clinical work (Tantam 2000).

Negative peer experiences: victimisation

A group of AS adolescents attending an intervention is likely to contain at least one if not more participants who are out of school. There are many reasons for their non-attendance but peer bullying and peer rejection are probably top of the list. Most of the group, probably all, will have been bullied in the past. Vulnerability of students with AS is high because of the nature of their social inter-action difficulties (Tantam 2000). The absence of empathy for others, lack of socio-emotional understanding of others, difficulty understanding peer non-verbal communication, all contribute to multiple misunderstandings between them and their peers. A recent Irish study showed that the type of bullying experienced by students with AS was different from that experienced by typical peers. Ridicule and social exclusion were the most common forms experienced, and rates of bullying were 25 times greater than experienced by typical peers (Lawlor, Harpur and James 2004).

The personal qualities that adolescents value in friends are exactly those that people with AS usually lack (Mobbs Henry *et al.* 1995). Their difficulties in initiating conversations and lack of interest in popular issues contribute to their social exclusion. A major protective factor against being bullied is to have some friends. A history of victimisation and poor social relations predicts the onset of emotional problems in adolescence. A consequence of young people not having friends is a higher incidence of depression. This condition is relatively common in AS adolescents. A depressive affect may lead to rejection by peers. The presence of mental health problems is likely to reduce the chance of making friends. Another factor that increases vulnerability to being bullied is being anxious or passive in the face of conflict. Being friendless increases the risk of being bullied and those that are persistently bullied are avoided by non-bullying peers. A cycle of victimisation is established that is difficult to escape. These adolescents need an immense amount of support to avoid school bullying. It is not possible to address bullying and halt it solely through a social interaction intervention. The school must deal with school bullying.

The experiences that many of these adolescents have had at the hands of their peers may have left them feeling depressed, anxious, angry and lonely. Some of these adolescents express suicidal thoughts. It is necessary to understand their expectations and motivation against this background in an intervention.

Intellectualisation: a common defence

Some points about the AS mindset are so important that they need repeating. People with AS often require a justification for a particular rule or statement before they will accept it. In discussion periods, providing justifications for the topic that is the subject for discussion may be challenging, satisfying or irksome. Nevertheless, it has to be done. One illustration of this is the resistance of those with AS to change. A therapist may be challenged by a response such as: 'Why do we need to learn about conversation anyway? Most people are dull and I couldn't be bothered talking to them.' That is a mouthful to confront, no doubt about that. How best to handle it? The wrong way is to say something like 'Well everyone else thinks it is important' or worse 'That's complete rubbish, I won't even bother to reply to it'. Responses that are more effective are based on:

- judging whether the participant is being oppositional and defiant

- implementing a conflict avoidance strategy (see 'banned phrase' later)

- replying calmly with an informed statement.

In the case at hand, an evolutionary justification for conversation and cooperation is worth invoking (survival interdependence between individual and group requires communication and cooperation to achieve basic life-enhancing goals such as acquiring food).

There is an old story about a group of rabbis who were invited to share a large pot of soup set in the middle of a circular table. Unfortunately, the spoons left out for the rabbis were so long that no one could turn the spoon back into his mouth. No one could feed himself. The rabbis sat there hungry for a long while trying to come up with a solution. Then, almost at once, they began to realise one by one that each could feed his neighbour. This is the value of cooperation.

Motivation torpor

What happens when the intervention does not meet expectations? There are no guarantees that the intervention will be successful. Confounding factors include the constitution of the participant, uneven delivery of the material, inappropriate management of the group, adolescents and/or parents are not sufficiently engaged, too many mismatched participants in the group and, finally, inadequate comprehension of the underlying principles.

Sometimes, a participant is not ready for group interaction. He may appear resistant when really his motivation is extremely low: so low in fact that sameness is less threatening than any slight explorations of change. In these cases, the participants' expectations are backward looking rather future oriented. The desire to reverse out of the session is overwhelming.

Colm attended the intervention having been through several social skills interventions and a range of schools. He was 15 years old and had been diagnosed with AS at the age of 9 years. His IQ was in the superior range and at one level this made his absence from school all the more upsetting. Colm's interests revolved solely around the computer. He was a pleasant young adolescent but presented as markedly timid and ill at ease in company. His eyes would frequently dart away from whoever was addressing him. His mother was supportive and made every effort to avail of whatever might help him. However, she remarked before he joined the intervention that she might not be able to persuade him to come along. Eventually, he did come but left after two sessions. It was not possible to coax him into returning.

In retrospect, Colm may have benefited from a pre-intervention course of therapy had resources been available. A 'pre-course' may have helped him develop adequate *foreknowledge* of what to expect and, analogous to a metal, he would have been tempered for the task. The conundrum is deciding just how much of a 'pre-course' is required before someone participates in any intervention. The nature of AS is that preparation for an abstract exercise may be perfectly acceptable to the individual concerned, but he or she may still flinch from a commitment to action in the company of others.

Anxiety management

The world of social interaction is often confusing, unpredictable, frustrating and frightening. People with AS are seen by others as socially naive and regularly subjected to ridicule and harassment. Probably the most commonly experienced emotions by people with AS are fear and anxiety. Any group interaction intervention with adolescents with AS has to include a regular module on anxiety management which addresses understandable initial anxiety within the group and inevitable anxiety in the outside world. Changes in routines are stressful for people with AS. General anxiety management strategies are outlined below and the group will need to be given regular reminders to regularly implement them:

- If you have a worry or feel upset, talk to someone you trust who understands you about any problems you may be having.

- Practise relaxation exercises daily. These can be taught within the group.

- Muscle relaxation exercises, breathing exercises or other meditative exercises can be practised both within and outside the group.

- Do enjoyable relaxing activities everyday.

- Engage in positive self-talk.

- Do some positive and useful act every day.

- Get 30 minutes of physical exercise every day.

- Avoid coffee.

- Prepare yourself as well as you can for new situations; e.g. Research a new school in advance, make a number of visits and get yourself orientated before you start there as a pupil.

A wide variety of relaxation techniques can help relieve muscle tension and 'racing heart' caused by excessive stress. The adolescents could be advised to incorporate one of the following two exercises into their everyday life: muscle relaxation and breathing exercises.

Muscle relaxation

You can do these exercises sitting up in a comfortable chair, or lying down. Remember to breathe in and out slowly and evenly. Breathe out as slowly as you can manage (obviously not to the point of discomfort):

1. Tense up your shoulders so they almost reach your ears. Hold them there as you count slowly to ten. Then let go and relax.

2. Pull your elbows into the sides of your body. Bend your arms upwards so your hands touch your shoulders, and then clench your fists as tightly as you can. Hold this position as you count slowly to ten and then let go and relax.

3. Tighten your stomach muscles. Hold as you count slowly to ten. Let go and relax.

4. Focus on your feet on the ground. Tighten your thigh muscles and curl your toes. Hold tightly as you count slowly to ten. Let go and relax.

5. Concentrate on your breathing. Take in a deep breath. Hold it for a few seconds and slowly let go. As you let go, loosen the muscles on your face and forehead, so your eyes and eyelids feel heavier. Gradually let your jaw slacken. Let your shoulders and stomach loosen. Let your arms and legs feel heavier.

6. Continue breathing slowly and evenly until you feel quiet, heavy and warm.

Breathing exercises

Breathing exercises can be practised several times per day. They can be practised before you go into a stressful situation, and you can continue them while in the situation to help you feel calmer. Taking deep breaths will help you manage panic attacks. The exercises are very straightforward and no one will notice you practising them. If you become fearful in a social situation, it will help if you remember to practise the following exercise in particular:

1. Breathe in slowly and deeply.

2. Count to five as you breathe in.

3. Hold your breath for a few seconds and then slowly count to five as you breathe slowly out.

4. The deeper you breathe in and the more slowly you breathe out, the more you will relax.

5. Do this six times, and if you still feel very anxious, do it again.

Psychiatric problems associated with Asperger syndrome

Many adolescents with Asperger syndrome also have psychiatric problems and some may have several (Ghaziuddin 2005). In the past, quite a number of people with AS came to the attention of health professionals because they presented with depression or anxiety problems in adolescence. It was only after careful assessment and treatment of the psychiatric condition that the underlying Asperger syndrome was revealed. The most common comorbidities are described briefly below.

Anxiety disorders

Anxiety can become extreme, and may manifest as an anxiety disorder. Anxiety disorders take a number of forms, which include:

- social anxiety disorder

- panic attacks

- generalised anxiety disorder

- obsessive compulsive disorder.

These conditions are very distressing and disruptive but it is important to remember that they can be treated.

Social anxiety disorder

Many adolescents with AS have had a difficult time socially in school. They often suffer considerable fear and anxiety. Anyone who has experienced being rebuffed, rejected, excluded or isolated in social situations understandably becomes very afraid and anxious about these experiences being repeated. Consequently, they may desire to avoid social situations as much as possible. Avoidance in turn leads to further social isolation which tends to worsen the situation. Social anxiety disorder is a common condition in people with AS. It can become overpowering if not addressed properly.

This condition often begins in adolescence. The central problem here is a fear of scrutiny by other people in comparatively small groups (as opposed to crowds). The individual feels he or she will act in a way that will be humiliating or embarrassing. This fear then leads on to feelings of anxiety, hand tremor, blushing, progressing to panic attacks in the feared social situation. These intense feelings of anxiety, if unresolved, result in avoidance of the situation. This avoidance then interferes with one's normal routine and academic and social functioning. When avoidance is extreme, it can lead to complete social isolation. A number of adolescents with social anxiety disorder are brought to mental health services because of refusal to attend school.

Panic attacks

Panic attacks are sudden feelings of intense fear and terror. Your heart beats very quickly and may feel as if it is pounding in your chest. Your hands may be shaking and you may be sweating. You feel overwhelmed by fear. You may have a pain in your stomach. You may believe you are seriously ill and about to die. Panic attacks are not uncommon among people with AS. New environments, new routines and strangers all exacerbate any fear of uncertainty.

Although an attack usually lasts only for a few minutes, most sufferers feel distressed for quite some time afterwards. Panic attacks can occur every time you are in a particular situation. The situation is a 'trigger'. However, panic attacks may happen suddenly for no apparent reason whatsoever. Sometimes panic attacks can occur in other illnesses, for example, depression. People who experience panic attacks often have other anxiety symptoms including obsessive compulsive disorder or generalised anxiety disorder. Frequently these are accompanied by depression.

What causes panic attacks?

Panic attacks can be triggered by stressful events such as not knowing what to do in a situation, being ridiculed by others, misunderstanding a social context, relationship breakdown, disappointments, the death of someone supportive, and other stressful incidents. There is some evidence that anxiety disorders also have a genetic component. However, the good news is that panic attacks can be successfully treated.

Generalised anxiety disorder

Communication is pretty much a multitasking affair. Lots of inputs from the environment have to be processed and are competing for your attention. Anyone with AS finds it extremely difficult to consciously focus on what other people are actually saying and on how and what they are communicating nonverbally. Trying to understand what is happening in a conversation and at the same time having to plan how to respond, and remember turn taking, can be overwhelming in certain contexts. Achieving some measure of social success can be very hard won. A minority of those with AS may be so afraid and anxious about their performance that they will be in a constant state of uncontrollable fear, worrying and anxiety. This is a condition called generalised anxiety disorder (GAD). It is a long-term condition which often persists for many years before diagnosis and treatment. GAD is an illness which interferes with everyday life. It has associated physical symptoms, just like anxiety. Someone who worries excessively about minor things, is tense most days and anxious most of the time is likely to have a generalised anxiety disorder. When worry, anxiety and tension persist for six months or more, they constitute a disorder. Symptoms of GAD include:

- nervousness or restlessness
- poor concentration
- irritable or depressed mood
- muscle tension
- disturbed sleep.

Many people with GAD also feel depressed about life and the cycle of anxiety that is their everyday experience. This condition can start in late adolescence and is more common in women than in men.

WHAT CAUSES GENERALISED ANXIETY DISORDER?

Research indicates that biological factors, family background and life experiences are important contributors to the triggering and maintenance of this condition. The communication difficulties of people with AS make them more vulnerable to developing this condition. The fear of committing a miscommunication can cause immense anxiety. Many sufferers report an increase in stressful positive or negative life events in the months or even years prior to the onset of the condition. This condition often coexists with other anxiety disorders, including alcohol and drug abuse problems. However, the point again to remember is that GAD is treatable, but you will need professional medical assistance.

Obsessive compulsive disorder

People with AS dislike departures from routines. Routines are reliable, predictable and certain. Some people may even develop symptoms of obsessive compulsive disorder (OCD) because of their attachment to routines. The performance of rituals is often a feature of OCD. This is a condition which usually begins in late childhood or adolescence. It affects between 1 to 2 per cent of the general population and is characterised by *obsessions* and *compulsions*. A recent study suggests its frequency among people with AS is much higher than previously suspected (Russell *et al.* 2005).

Obsessions are unwanted, repetitive, intrusive thoughts. The commonest are listed below:

- fear of contamination by dirt or germs
- being overly concerned about symmetry or the orderly arrangement of things
- fear of aggressive impulses
- worrying about unusual sexual thoughts
- having doubts about things they know they should not be worried about.

Compulsions are urges to carry out rituals. Different rituals that people perform include:

- washing and hand washing
- checking
- measuring
- counting
- hoarding
- need to ask or confess.

A ritual helps relieve the fear and anxiety created by obsessive thoughts. Rituals can be very time consuming. They can interfere with all aspects of your life. For instance, some people may take many hours to complete all their rituals in the morning before leaving the house. A simple five-minute task may take hours to complete once all the rituals are observed.

John was diagnosed with AS at age 10. After changing to another secondary school at age 15 he began to develop a number of rituals which he performed before leaving the house in the morning. These included repeated hand washing and teeth brushing, packing his schoolbag and checking it repeatedly, and closing all the room doors in a particular order. The packing of the schoolbag then started at night and could take up to two hours to complete, which interfered with his sleep. At school he would only take notes on a certain type of paper and use certain pens for different subjects. The school were concerned about his lateness for school, checking behaviour in school and the non-completion of his homework. They notified his parents, who then took John to the family doctor. He recommended referral to a psychiatrist, who in turn diagnosed John with OCD and prescribed medication, engaged him in a course of cognitive behavioural therapy in conjunction with his parents and worked out a management plan with the family and school. John was seen regularly by the school counsellor to help with problems at school. The symptoms gradually receded.

John's OCD is not uncommon. However, his capacity to be an effective student was rapidly disappearing. Among people that like routines OCDs are noticeable. However, if obsessions and rituals begin to overpower someone's life the help of a medical doctor should be sought.

Treatments for anxiety disorders

There are a number of different treatment approaches for anxiety disorders. These include different types of psychotherapy and/or medication. All of these treatments will be enhanced by the regular practice of relaxation and tension-reducing exercises. It is important to seek a therapist who is familiar with nonverbal communication problems and has an understanding of autistic spectrum disorders.

Psychotherapy services are increasingly accessible. Cognitive behavioural psychotherapy can help treat anxiety disorders. Psychodynamic psychotherapy where there is a focus on the action part of the self may be beneficial. Cognitive behavioural therapy can be appealing to some people with AS. However, psychoanalytic psychotherapy focusing on the unconscious is not recommended.

Medication is a very useful treatment for anxiety disorders. Different types of medication are given for short-term and long-term treatment of these conditions. Many people with disabling anxiety problems find that medication makes a substantial difference to their quality of life. The most commonly prescribed medications for these disorders are called SSRIs, e.g. Prozac. They have positive effects on anxiety, obsessive compulsive disorder, social phobia and depression.

These medications can also be used to help relieve some of the obsessional features of AS.

Depression

Depression is a relatively common phenomenon in adolescents with AS. Some studies have indicated that there may be a genetic link between autistic spectrum disorder (including AS) and depressive illness. Many become depressed as a result of negative social interactions with siblings, parents and peers. Victimisation by peers is a common experience. Increased self-consciousness of adolescence, increasing awareness of difference from peers and lack of company all combine to make a reactive depressive cocktail. Depression can also occur for all the reasons that affect everyone else, such as loss, disappointment, humiliation, etc.

Depression is characterised by a persistently negative view of the self, the world and the future. In adolescents this may present as irritability, loss of enjoyment in life, sleeping too much and either undereating or overeating. There may be suicidal feelings, ideas, intentions and actions. The treatment of choice for these adolescents is psychotherapy, generally of the cognitive/behavioural variety, combined if necessary with antidepressant medication.

Some adolescents may have what is called endogenous depression where they may have sleep and appetite disturbances, diurnal mood variation and possibly an array of somatic complaints. There may be no emotionally triggering events. Antidepressant treatment is usually the treatment of choice combined with psychotherapy.

It may be the case that some adolescents with AS are too depressed to be involved in a group and may need to be treated for depression prior to joining a social interaction therapy group. Sometimes people may feel so depressed that it is not possible to engage in psychotherapy. At this point they may need their doctor to prescribe antidepressant medication. This medication is not addictive. Depressed people have to be patient as this medication does not work immediately.

In some cases, admission to an adolescent psychiatric unit may be necessary. This may be necessary if outpatient treatment was insufficient, if the person is persistently suicidal, has made suicidal acts or is thought to be a risk to themselves or to others. Admission is a very last resort however. It is important to remember that the world of the depressed person is a very different world from that of most of us. On these occasions, depression is like a lens that twists things out of focus. When this happens, the depressed person may not understand that the various services are trying to help.

Suicidal thoughts and behaviour

Many children with AS tend to talk openly about death and suicide. This becomes more dangerous in adolescence as around the age of puberty the rate of suicidal acts tends to increase markedly. These suicidal acts are often in response to the overwhelming demands of the social world and bullying. Some adolescents have attempted suicide because a peer told them "Go kill yourself" in anger.

Expression of suicidal ideation and intent cannot be ignored. Parents will need to be informed if participants express suicidal ideation or describe plans for suicide or suicidal acts.

One psychiatrist's experience is that a helpful response to expressed suicidal ideation in AS is to say: 'It is not a good idea to try and kill yourself. Some people who have tried have been unsuccessful and have ended up being brain damaged and that would not be good for you' (Gillberg 2002, p.52). Suicide is a dangerous experiment. Suicide should be identified as an illogical choice as no one has a copy of tomorrow's newspaper and no one can predict the future. Many people who feel suicidal one day may feel quite differently the next.

Attention deficit hyperactivity disorder

Many people with AS also have problems with attention. Sometimes they may seem not to be paying any attention to the outside world at all and may then demonstrate evidence to the contrary. In some cases they hyperfocus on their specific area of interest to the exclusion of all other interests. Some may become more inattentive because they are under stress and on these occasions it is worth enquiring of parents if anything untoward has happened or is troubling the adolescent.

Some may have the type of attention deficit seen in attention deficit hyperactivity disorder (ADHD) (combined type) where inattention occurs with hyperactivity and impulsivity. These can manifest in the group by relentless interrupting, off-topic comments, inattentiveness and hyperactivity. Others may have a predominantly inattentive problem that may meet the diagnostic criteria for attention deficit disorder (ADD). Some modifications of these behaviours can occur by:

- weekly repetition of group rules

- the use of previously agreed visual and verbal cues/reminders to members who tend to be disruptive due to ADHD

- by asking parents on the day of the group to remind the young person about trying to pay attention in the group.

Sometimes the level of inattentiveness, impulsivity or hyperactivity may be very difficult to contain in the group setting. If the level of disruption caused by this type of behaviour is interfering with the other group members progressing, the situation needs to be assessed. An unacceptably high level of ADHD-type behaviour should be brought to the parents' attention and they should be asked to have the situation assessed by the adolescent's psychiatrist. If inattention, impulsivity or hyperactive behaviour are manifested on a sustained basis, it may be the case that stimulant medication would be helpful. It is worth remembering that if the groups are held in the evening some stimulant medications may be wearing off at this time and may need readjusting. In extreme cases, in the interests of other group members a young person may need to be withdrawn from the group for a time to allow the inattentiveness to be treated.

Oppositional defiance

Where the AS participant is oppositionally defiant and persistently engages in negative interaction, a helpful strategy is to:

- remind the person to produce constructive comment

- ignore provocative and negative output

- respond with neutral statements such as 'I appreciate your point of view, but I think there is an alternative point of view as well.'

Avoid confrontation with this type of adolescent. Due to past social rejection, he or she may feel more secure with a hostile response. Of course, a therapist may feel disparaged and undermined in this situation. It can happen that he or she may unwittingly react in a hostile manner, which only serves to justify the adolescent's resistance to change.

It is important to bear in mind that a display of social negativity in those with AS frequently masks profound social distress and emotional confusion. A display of negative cognitions, while not explained by current theories of autism, is quite common. People with AS are frequently quite frightened of change – any change in behaviour or routine. The therapist is charged with helping the adolescents to imagine things differently. Managing these participants effectively within the group requires patience and, most importantly, respect. If necessary, a private word out of earshot of the group may be helpful. Gradually, these adolescents can be 'brought around' by:

- using neutral statements

- enforcing the constructive comment rule

- soliciting their opinions actively when alternatives to other positions are required.

Other conditions

TICS AND TOURETTE'S SYNDROME

Tics are very common in AS. One Swedish study found that 80 per cent of people with AS had tics. It was also found that over 10 per cent of schoolchildren with AS also had Tourette's syndrome.

RARER CONDITIONS IN AS

The two conditions described briefly below tend to occur in about 1 per cent of the population. There is no evidence that they are any more common in people with AS than in the general population.

SCHIZOPHRENIA

This is a long-term condition that tends to start in late adolescence or early adulthood. It is characterised by hallucinations, delusions, thought disorder, social withdrawal and personality deterioration.

MANIC DEPRESSIVE ILLNESS

Manic depressive illness (or bipolar disorder) is characterised by episodes of depression alternating with episodes of hypomania or (more severely) mania. Manic episodes manifest in increased talkativeness, difficulties concentrating, reduced need and desire for sleep, overspending, engaging in reckless irresponsible behaviours uncharacteristic over-sociability, inflated self-esteem, grandiosity and often greatly increased sexual activity.

Conclusions: in or out of the group?

Problematic behaviours can arise in a group setting that may require short-term withdrawal of a participant if not outright removal. Before obtaining parental consent and participant consent, it is mandatory to have in place a procedure for dealing with problematic behaviours. This procedure should be fully explained to all parties. If a participant is disruptive, aggressive or continually oppositional, their behaviour can inhibit participation by others at an attentional level and in terms of behavioural inputs.

Christopher joined a social skills group at the age of 13 years. He had been diagnosed with Asperger syndrome at the age of seven years. School support and various out-treatment services were provided in the intervening years. At each of the seven sessions he attended Christopher's behaviour and verbal reactions were exceptionally oppositional. He was a most unwilling participant in almost every group activity and voiced negative and distorted cognitions whenever the opportunity arose. He would not participate in roleplay, tending to dismiss the opportunities for rehearsal and feedback as 'boring', 'crap', 'ridiculous' and 'unrealistic'. He was also 'happy with his AS' and professed no interest in changing. Eventually, after consultation with his parents, Christopher withdrew from the group as there was a consensus that his behaviour and disposition were inhibiting participation by the others.

Once quarantining (giving a participant a period of time out of the group activities) had failed to produce the required cognitive restructuring or change in behaviour, the only alternative was to postpone further group involvement and refer the participant to the relevant individual therapist. Christopher's story is interesting as the therapist involved mentioned that this was the first time in 15 years that the withdrawal of a participant was required to stabilise the group. Cases like Christopher's are relatively uncommon, but they also confirm the puzzling tension between sameness and difference in AS. In most situations participants can be managed effectively and their participation obtained.

The compelled withdrawal of a participant should not be treated lightly. It can have a profound impact by reinforcing negative and distorted cognitions (thoughts) about the self and world. 'I told you it wouldn't work. Why did you force me to go? It's all crap anyway' are commonly expressed reactions in these cases. Furthermore, parents may be very resistant to the withdrawal proposal. Unless they have consented to the procedure in advance, an unsatisfactory situation will remain unresolved. In problematic cases, the degree to which oppositional behaviour (hostility) may mask a depressive illness should not be ignored. The incidence of depression among AS adolescents is quite high. Any concerns about a participant's behaviour or mood should always be discussed in the first instance with the parents to determine if a psychiatric review is necessary.

8 Session Plans and Materials

In this chapter we outline several sample session plans. These should be sufficient to guide the development of a complete set tailored to specific intervention needs and resources. Earlier chapters, especially Chapter 6, deal with broad methodological and theoretical issues. Here we focus on the common factors that inform the possibility of change in a group. Once these are identified, particular components of session are presented.

Common factors in interventions

Experience across the globe reveals that many interventions that should 'work' either fail completely or are at best uneven in their efficacy. Asperger syndrome does not have a complete medical explanation. Many of its more subtle but profound manifestations are still being uncovered. However, a range of common behaviours, cognitive and emotional 'styles' are accepted as the factors that should be subject to change within any therapeutic model. Until scientific knowledge improves, consolidation of all these factors and more besides into a single therapeutic model will be a matter of best practice, preference – and disagreement. Our approach to interventions is plural. The issue is not whether 'other' interventions have something to offer, but how best to make use of what they offer vis-à-vis challenges faced by AS adolescents. Commenting on the dilemmas facing therapists torn between following a particular model and working with what works for them, one therapist noted:

As with most practitioners, the usefulness of doing what worked took precedence over theoretical purity. I began to borrow techniques from a variety of models to fit the student and situation with favourable results. These real-world experiences, combined with the futile search for the best model from the literature, convinced me that no single model is adequate in explaining and treating the wide variety of people and problems encountered by practitioners. One nagging question remained: How can treatment models that appear very different in theoretical orientation and technique yield similar outcomes? Enter common factors. (Murphy 1999, p.362)

The common factors, the ingredients, that contribute to change as follows (adapted slightly from Murphy 1999):

1. Participant's personal strengths and resources.

2. Relationship with therapist in terms of perceived understanding and respect.

3. Expectancy that a participant has of the therapy and the possibility of change.

4. Model or technique employed by the therapist.

Making the best use of these common factors, mobilising them, is the basis for successful outcomes. Although Murphy's advice is not derived from explicit involvement with Asperger syndrome adolescents, it is based on experience of adolescents in school settings. It contains a plea for tolerance of approaches; A plea that we are sympathetic to, provided a therapist extends the four-factor list above to include a fifth factor. This fifth factor is the set of issues distinctively germane to Asperger syndrome:

- current theoretical and scientific insights on the condition

- pragmatic capacities

- discourse skills

- socio-emotional regulation and recognition

- prosodic problems.

What this all means in practice is that session plans, their content, structure and outcome emphasis are best adopted as heuristics, with the aid of the five common factors, to help form, deliver and manage an intervention (Figure 8.1).

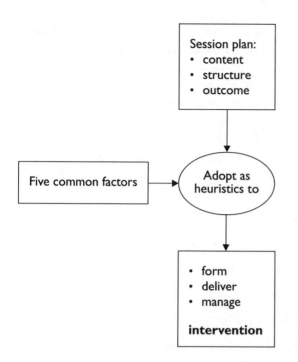

Figure 8.1 Session plans adopted as heuristics, with the aid of the five common factors, to form, deliver and manage an intervention

Resources and expectations

Resource allocation is another common concern. It is not part of an intervention in content terms, but it is an organisational reality. Service providers usually have one question on their mind: How long will it take? It is a reasonable question. Therapists may be unable to invest the time in administration, delivery, feedback and training if there is no proportionality between these tasks and similar treatments for other childhood and adolescent disorders. Purely in terms of allocating resources, interventions are bounded by time. It is impossible to state categorically the number of hours sufficient for a group with AS due to both the heterogeneity of the condition and the profound difficulties experienced by those with it. Much depends on the triangle of relationships among group characteristics, resources and individual therapist skills. There is no convenient response to these concerns. Tailoring an intervention for groups and specific participants within groups is inevitable given the heterogeneity of the condition. A great deal depends on the alliance, collaboration and relationship between participants and therapists. Therapists must demonstrate to participants (parents and adolescents) more than a competence with the intervention. They must show that they believe in it. If a therapist lacks confidence in the intervention, this will be transmitted to the group.

People with Asperger syndrome like a rationale for decisions and actions. They also like consistency and predictability. To develop trust during the early phase of an intervention, these preferences should be harnessed. At all stages of the intervention, justifications for decisions and strategies should be offered when requested by participants. As group collaboration and interaction improves, issues responding to unpredictability can be gradually explored. At all stages, a session should express and reference:

- *structure* – creates sense of predictability

- *rules* – establishes boundaries and expectations

- *relaxation* – learning cannot occur without it

- *humour* – reducing anxiety builds confidence

- *supervision* – management of behaviour through rules

- *security* – safe from ridicule and emotional injury

- *esteem* – everyone is valued

- *environment* – natural environment of participants, e.g. school

- *feedback* – constructive comment on participation.

Change is at the heart of all interventions. Acknowledging and working with rather than against a participant's expectations is important. At the beginning of the intervention, an assessment of participants' expectation should be undertaken. Soliciting the expectations of participants in the beginning and periodically throughout the intervention will help tailor the content, delivery and feedback.

Listening to the participants, helping them tell their stories and compare experiences with each other, serves to create common ground in the group. These processes also help tailor the intervention to their needs and expectations. Trying to bring the group around to considering what they want from the intervention and how they see themselves achieving this are useful strategies for probing their self-understanding and expectations. Typical elicitation questions include:

- What to you want to get out of coming here?

- What do you hope (think) will be different after these sessions?

- What one or two things do you really want to change in your life?

- What small change will show you these sessions are working out?

Questions should be short, concrete and pitched in simple language. It is tempting to assume that the expectations of those with AS are obvious. They are not. AS adolescents may appear to want the same goals as typical peers, but the possibility of subtle differences should be considered. The therapist should elaborate their goals to ensure:

- clarity

- agreement

- eliminate social bias in responses.

> When Greg came to a group, he proclaimed firmly that he wanted to make friends with people in his class. The therapist helped him elaborate this goal and discovered that he wanted friends because *he was being bullied*. If he could only make friends with the bullies, his life would be better – Greg's reasoning.

Greg's desire to make friends is very common. It also reveals a skewed understanding of friendship as a state of not being harassed by peers. Many people with Asperger syndrome have a distorted grasp of friendship. They do not understand friendship as either a process involving affiliation, intersubjectivity, sharing or social identity formation.

Adolescence is a stressful experience for everyone. The typical adolescent is experimenting with independence from parents, 'get away from me', while at the same time needing them 'look after me'. The adolescent with Asperger syndrome faces a dilemma here. Emotional immaturity means that dependency upon parents is greater than among peers, fuelling resentment. While at the same time, the option of moving closer to peers is often denied. This situation is at the heart of their difficulties in adolescence. It is essential that an intervention should keep this understanding to the forefront of all activities. The next question is how to deal with it.

Session plans for the intervention

A typical schedule of sessions follows the format shown in Table 8.1. A few points should be borne in mind when looking over the session plans.

Table 8.1 Typical schedule of sessions	
Session no.	**Group**
1	Parents
2–5	Adolescents
6	Parents
7–11	Adolescents
12	Parents
13–19	Adolescents
20	Parents
21–25	Adolescents
26	Parents

First, in the interests of readability and space details, content has been trimmed. Elaborations in the initial sessions give sufficient insights into the structures of succeeding sessions. Second, the intervention is designed to start slowly and gradually accelerate in complexity. At around session 12, the group should be confident enough to take on robust role plays. However, some of the role plays will need to be adjusted for age. Each role play has an associated set of pragmatic capacities and discourse skills. The list is not exhaustive in every case and will need to be modelled with the group. It is preferable that the therapist models a solution and leaves it for exploration within the group. Third, 'party games' should be played at the end of sessions, if time permits. Finally, in practice it may not be possible to get through each role play in a session, nor cover each scenario. That is fine. Role plays may need to extend over several sessions to ensure appropriate modelling. We constantly emphasis that the focus is less on 'getting through' the material and more on checking that the participants are making progress. The material should be adapted in the light of the five factors.

Supplementary support sessions, 'booster' sessions, could be offered at staggered intervals after the completion of the main intervention. We do not provide a structure for these sessions here. In what follows we give a brief outline of each session. The therapist needs to expand the material in the light of the five factors mentioned in this chapter.

Session 1: Parents' introduction

This is an information session. Parents receive information about the intervention and are allowed time to digest it. A parent may prefer to take away any printed materials and return with a decision in a few days. That is perfectly reasonable. One way to lessen the information overload for the therapist is to encourage parents to read about Asperger syndrome.

The intervention is about developing and enhancing a broad range of pragmatic communication capacities in the adolescents (and the parents). For people who have never encountered the term before, defining *pragmatics* can seem a bit daunting. The simplest definition is that pragmatics refers to what we need to know before we use language effectively in social interactions. The objectives for this session are as follows:

1. Introduce the intervention to the parents.

2. Provide a description of Asperger syndrome.

3. Explain the significance of social interaction in adolescence.

4. Refer to the pragmatic rating scale when illustrating AS difficulties.

5. Indicate the parental role in the intervention.

6. Encourage parents to ask questions.

7. Solicit their consent to be involved.

Give parents contact times should they wish to discuss issues outside the standard group setting. These contact times should be introduced as contact rules with parents. Establishing boundaries requires clear setting of rules of contact.

Session 2: Adolescents' introduction

Every adolescent session focuses on developing and enhancing the following topics:

- relaxation

- self-confidence and self-esteem

- communication and social interaction capacities and skills.

Each session has a *set structure* as shown in Table 8.2 (assume this is part of all the sessions – we will flag any departures).

Table 8.2 Structure of adolescent sessions

Activity	Goal
Relaxation exercises	Anxiety reduction
Introduce *banned phrases* rule	Constructive criticism and positive comment are more encouraging than disparagement.
Introduce oneself by name	Auditory memory issue. Learning that knowing another's name is expected in peer settings. Can be eased as the group coheres.
Previous week's tales: participants tell about something that happened *to them* in the previous week that involved peers.	Talking about oneself publicly. Sharing personal experiences. Providing common ground for conversation. Must be time managed.
Theme/topic	Show structure: name it and model it.
Rehearsal and role play	Develops social problem solving skills.
Practice work for the adolescent	Encourages social interaction between sessions.
Practice work for the *adolescent and parent – will vary between sessions*	Involves parents in the intervention and serves to remind them of its purpose.

The introductory period embraces the first two sessions with the adolescents. The participants introduce themselves to the group. The therapist models the desired interactions making sure to get each participant's attention. Additionally, the banned phrases rule must be presented and explained. This rule states that only constructive criticism and positive comments are allowed. It is a crucial *always on* rule. The group could be encouraged to make a list of likely offending phrases in this session, but it may be more useful to 'get through' this session and revisit it in the next session.

Session 3: Eliciting expectations

Begin with a welcome, followed by the relaxation exercises, and state the rules for the group.

Big Rule: EVERYONE PARTICIPATES. No one may be excused participation. Get the group to state the banned phrases rule.

Introduce one another by name.

TASK

What happened to each participant last week? Use this to reinforce name recall. Note where each person is sitting and remember to shift them in the next session.

Describe session structure.

TOPIC: ELICIT PARTICIPANTS' EXPECTATIONS

Model and encourage cross-comparison:

- Signal to each participant that they all have something in common such as school. Even those not currently attending school can complete this exercise based on their last school.

- Encourage the sharing of experiences about school and its challenges. In turn, this inculcates an attitude that being in school is the norm, it is expected.

Session 4: Talking about Asperger syndrome

> Begin with a welcome, followed by the relaxation exercises, and state the rules for the group.
>
> Big Rule: EVERYONE PARTICIPATES. No one may be excused participation. Get the group to state the banned phrases rule.
>
> Introduce one another by name.
>
> TASK
>
> What happened to each participant last week? Use this to reinforce name recall. Note where each person is sitting and remember to shift them in the next session.
>
> Describe session structure.

TOPIC: ASPERGER SYNDROME – WHAT IT MEANS TO ME

Everyone in the group needs to know that they have a diagnosis of AS in order for this session to proceed. The therapist can lead off with: 'I want you to talk about Asperger syndrome and what it means to each of you. I want each of you to tell me, and the group, when you first found out you had AS and what you felt at the time. Okay?'

Activity	Goal
Ask each member to describe *to the others*: (a) when he or she was first diagnosed; (b) their reaction.	Encourages (a) identification with others through common experiences; (b) helps form a group identity.
Ask the group whether they have any experiences in common. Try to steer the discussion towards: (a) identifying common elements of experience; (b) followed by common reactions.	Focus on sharing experiences as helping people get to know each other. The group will have many problems in common. Perspective-taking exercise.

Ask each member to picture *for one of his neighbours* how someone without AS might understand it.	Exploratory point of view exercise acknowledging the typical adolescent's perspective.
Ask the group what seems to be working for other adolescents but not as well for those with AS.	This is building up to presenting ideas about communication and social interaction expectations.
Emphasise to the group that *it is okay to be different.* Cite famous historical thinkers as role models.	Reassurance that difference does not always imply disability. Asperger syndrome has strengths and weaknesses.
Model several communicative acts: e.g. greeting and thanking among adolescents. Get two members from the group to role play the acts afterwards.	This is an observation exercise for: (a) the therapist; and (b) the group. Focus is on getting someone else's attention – catching their eye.
Conclude by asking the group whether this session was a high note or a low note for them.	Purpose is to probe their relaxedness in the setting.

Session 5: Other people and Asperger syndrome

Begin with a welcome, followed by the relaxation exercises, and state the rules for the group.

Big Rule: EVERYONE PARTICIPATES. No one may be excused participation. Get the group to state the banned phrases rule.

Introduce one another by name.

TASK

What happened to each participant last week? Use this to reinforce name recall. Note where each person is sitting and remember to shift them in the next session.

Describe session structure.

TOPIC: ASPERGER SYNDROME – WHAT IT MEANS TO OTHERS

In the previous session, the group explored the diagnosis of Asperger syndrome and what it meant to each of them. In this session they will be asked to explore tentatively the perspectives of others such as adolescent peers. This session builds on the work in the previous session using a role play involving a game of four people. Three is the minimum number for this game to have any force.

Activity	Goal
Role play involving four adolescents from the group, three of whom have been coached in the rules. The remaining adolescent participates without knowing the rules. His task is to work them out (infer them).	The game is a microcosm of the interaction confusion faced by people with AS. It encourages attention to others, especially their nonverbal body language. The game embraces the principle that all communication is an invitation to inference.
A variation on the game involves giving turns at the table to all the non-coached members of the group.	Broadens group participation and turntaking opportunities. It also encourages shared experiences.

ACTIVITY: FIVE-MINUTE GAME

The role play is based around three or four participants labelling hand positions correctly. The twist is that only three of the participants know the rules. Additional excitement and mystery can be added if three players are taken aside so that only they know the rules. The game can then be played with several members of the group in turn playing the role of the person trying to figure out the rules. *We recommend that only volunteers be accepted for this role – a therapist should lead off as a model of rule ignorance.*

Players sit around a table and are allowed three hand positions: (1) one hand or elbow on the table, called '*one up one down*'; (2) two hands or elbows on the table, called '*two up two down*' (3) no hands or elbows on the table, called '*two down*'. Players are only allowed to say '*I'm two up two down*', and so forth. The therapist has to judge whether the 'outsider' is robust enough for the role. It is important to ensure that the play is good humoured, respectful and not anxiety provoking. The session should conclude with a debriefing of the group about their own experiences with their peers.

The point of the activity is that it is only when we understand the rules of the game can we participate effectively. These experiences must be related to intersubjectivity. It is worthwhile now asking the participants to identify what they could have done differently on those occasions to get a better outcome. Their replies should be steered towards whether a better understanding of other people would have helped, and what would that might consist of. Permanent probing of reciprocity and peer expectations is required.

The game is a microcosm of the social experience of many people on the autistic spectrum. Interaction is taking place between others but the AS person does not comprehend the rules or operates with an incomplete set. Exhortations to 'get on with it', despite how ridiculous they sound, are experienced by many people with AS. This role play explores the importance of rules to other people and the need to pay careful attention to others' actions and words in framing interactions.

Session 6: Parents again

This session has several purposes:

- giving feedback on the adolescents in the previous sessions
- eliciting feedback from the parents
- addressing any concerns.

Activity	Goal
Ask parents to list examples of situations where the *banned phrases* rule was applied.	Persuade them of the importance in monitoring family communication styles.
Note feedback that parents believe is related to an intervention effect.	• Data collection • Indication of parental engagement with the intervention.
Describe any social effects questionnaires and answer questions about their use.	Introduce parents to the process of evaluation and their role within it.
Suggest a social calendar to the parents and ask them to draw up their own.	• Stimulate within-group contacts between adolescents • Prepare for transference of abilities to external world.

NOTES FOR THE THERAPIST

Some parents may resist 'firming up' dates in the social calendar. It is best if: (a) they can be encouraged to reach a decision within the session period; (b) give a date when such a decision will be reached and communicated. In general, it is preferable for one parent (or perhaps two) to become the coordinator of this process at least until the parents become comfortable with each other. Suggesting to the parents that they select a coordinator for liaison purposes is a sensible move.

Session 7: Reciprocity and turn taking
TOPIC: RECIPROCITY AND TURN TAKING I

Introduce the group to the *anthropologist metaphor*. Discuss with them a scenario where they have been shipwrecked on an island inhabited by people unfamiliar with their speech and customs. The group has to work out strategies for communicating their needs to the natives. Everyone must participate and it is best if tasks are parcelled out on an individual level. One person is assigned to communicate water needs, another must persuade the island people to provide food, and yet another must convey that they need help to leave the island. This exercise can be made more complicated by placing constraints on the use of language and encouraging only gesture. However, as this is a preliminary exercise it is best not to overcomplicate it. The exercise can be revisited.

Activity	Goal
Ask the group to explain the work of an anthropologist briefly.	Preparatory stimulation of frame of reference for the topic.
Explain reciprocity and turn taking in terms of their functions in social interaction.	Clarification of objective and an opportunity for them to raise questions.
Ask them to picture themselves as a group stranded on the island, and then begin the exploration.	Stimulate thinking about communication strategies and help them to practise several which involve nonverbal communication.
Invite them to conclude with a recapitulation of the important points and identify what has been learned.	Test of learning and comprehension. Also it is an opportunity to discuss real-world transference.
Give the group the questions as part of preparation for learning transference. Ask each to write out his or her answers and return with them at the next session.	Learning and comprehension exercise. It is important to encourage an understanding of communication as a social activity.

NOTES FOR THE THERAPIST

There are two versions of this theme. In the first case, each adolescent is asked to imagine that he or she is stranded among the island people. In the second version, the group as a whole is stranded and must coordinate its interactions with the natives to be effective. Depending on the size of the group, one section can act as island people. Alternatively, the therapist(s) can take this role. Modelling of nonverbal discourse skills by the therapist will be required.

Session 8: Active listening – reciprocity and turn taking 2
TOPIC: ACTIVE LISTENING – RECIPROCITY AND TURN TAKING 2

At this stage the group (most members) will have been practising what will be explicitly explored in this session, namely active listening. This is an opportunity to point out to each of them just how good their active listening has been, and to give examples of where it 'paid off' in the various role plays.

Activity	Goal
Ask the group to differentiate between *hearing and listening – is the latter important and why?*	Create frame of reference for the topic.
Give examples of peer listening contexts, e.g. school, study sessions, playground.	Focus attention on concrete situations of use.
Ask members of the group to role play a hearing context and a listening context.	Stimulate thinking about attention to others.
Ask members of the group to give examples of when active listening would have benefited them in the past.	Encourage reflection on the process in the context of actual rather than hypothetical experience.
Discuss advantages in active listening.	Make benefits explicit.
Invite members to model consequences of failing to actively listen to peers.	Experiment in perspective taking.
Encourage the group to critique their own performances.	Reinforce active listening as intrinsic to communication as a social activity.

At the end of the session, ask the participants to bring their favourite item to the next session. The item can be an object of clothing, a book, music CD, in fact, almost anything except animals.

Session 9: Conversation – initiation and maintenance I
TOPIC: INITIATING AND MAINTAINING CONVERSATION I

The purpose of this session is to enhance the quality of an interaction by focusing on what is in common between two people – in this case, the common item is clearly visible. Participants have brought along something they like. Encourage each of them to discuss it by (a) describing it; (b) stating why it is appealing. Next, each person's neighbour is requested to discuss the item in terms of its appeal for the other person.

Yes/no answers are not sufficient. Each reply to a question must be a sentence. Second, because each participant is bringing a favourite item, there is a risk that he or she may talk at length and violate the active listening rules. Third, turn taking must be monitored closely. Finally, a list of useful stock phrases that will invite others to give feedback is explained to the group. It does not have to be exhaustive. The list can be expanded in later sessions. Typical examples are:

- 'Stop me if I am boring you'

- 'I know I go on a bit when I talk about [favourite hobby]'

- 'I find that interesting, do you?'

Activity	Goal
Ask a member of the group to describe his or her favourite item.	Topic introduction.
Ask the person to the right of the first speaker to question him or her about their favourite item.	Conversation development.
Invite some members of the group to role play an ineffective version of the scenario below.	Stimulate comprehension of 'bad' conversational scripts. Focus on negative consequences for AS adolescent.
Invite other members of the group to role play the effective version of the scenario below.	Stimulate a comparative analysis and comprehension of properties of good social scripts. Focus on positive consequences for AS adolescent.
Give the group a list of stock phrases they can use to help them solicit feedback from peers.	Learning to solicit feedback on one's social interaction performances.

SCENARIO FOR ROLE PLAY

A group of teenagers in the same class is talking causally about a new computer game that has come out. Another teenager interrupts to talk about his favourite topic, which happens to be computers and computer games. He talks at length and eventually the group drift off.

How can he talk about his area of interest and avoid the negative reactions of peers?

NOTES FOR THE THERAPIST

The modelled solution should emphasise the use of stock phrases to cue turn taking: for example, 'I know I go on a bit about computers', 'Stop me if I am boring you', 'I just want to make two points and then you can ask.'

Session 10: Conversation – initiation and maintenance 2
TOPIC: INITIATING AND MAINTAINING CONVERSATION 2

This is a continuation of the previous session. To aid retention it should follow a similar structure. The purposes are to explore conversation initiation and topic maintenance. It is highly likely that the role play of the last session remained incomplete and even unsatisfactory. This is an opportunity to revisit and refine the lessons learnt from the last session. If the topic is unappealing and a fresh one is required, something historical may be substituted, for example World War II.

EXPECTATION VIOLATION

This is a point for exploration with the group. What happens when our expectations of another's interactions are violated? How do we react? How do we feel? Imagine staff in a takeaway restaurant completing an order with 'Have a crap day' rather than the expected 'Have a nice day'. Why do we feel there is something wrong here? How do we react? What do we think about the other person's behaviour?

Activity	Goal
Ask the group to describe or recall what was covered in the last session.	Topic introduction.
Ask each person for an example of a helpful stock phrase.	Conversation development.
Invite some members of the group to role play an ineffective version of the scenario.	Stimulate comprehension of 'bad' conversational scripts.
Invite others to critique it.	Comprehension exercise.
Select others to 'do it' as they imagine typical adolescents would.	Perspective taking; exploration of other peers' expectations.
Conclude with a group critique of the topic.	Learning and experience-sharing exercise.

NOTES FOR THE THERAPIST

This type of session should encourage spontaneous interactions within the group. It is important in these situations to keep members of the group alert when others are interacting. Inattentive participants will quickly lose the thread and find themselves confused when asked to be involved. Any explanation of strategies or skills should reference the importance of peer interaction expectations.

Session 11: Conversation – judging others' intentions
TOPIC: JUDGING OTHERS' INTENTIONS

The objective is to explore conversation initiation and response with unfamiliar peers. An unfamiliar peer is defined as a teenager whom a participant has never interacted with before, but recognises – possibly. For instance, the teenager could attend another school but hangs out at the same chess club. The teenager might hang around with other teenagers that a participant knows from school. The therapist should use the session to explore how members of the group reach judgements about peers. It is not a question of deciding that their judgements are right or wrong, more one of guiding them towards making safe judgements.

The scenario for the role play has an unfamiliar peer offer an item for sale to another peer (the 'teenager') in the setting of a takeaway restaurant. Is the unfamiliar peer genuine and trustworthy? Is he a smooth talking petty crook? How can one decide between these opposites? If one cannot decide, what is the safest interaction strategy to adopt? Underline to the group that whatever 'interaction recipes' are worked out for this scenario and similar ones may not always be successful. Sometimes one just has to get out quick!

Activity	Goal
Ask the group to describe and recall what was covered in the last session.	Recapitulation of main points.
Introduce the idea of conversing with unfamiliar peers and ask for examples.	Topic introduction.
Invite some members of the group to role play an ineffective version of the scenario.	Stimulate comprehension of 'bad' conversational scripts.
Select another group to 'do it' as they imagine typical adolescents would.	Perspective taking; exploration of other peers' expectations.
Conclude with a group critique of the topic: (a) the offer is morally sound; (b) the offer is morally unsound; (c) I am not sure.	Explore judgement formation regarding other peers. Introduce idea of behaviour appropriate to context.

SCENARIO FOR ROLE PLAY

> A teenager is in a queue in a pizza takeaway. Another teenager that he does not know offers him a Discman. The device appears to be in mint condition. The stranger says he was given it as a present but since he already has one, he wants to sell it. He is looking for half the shop price for the item.

How does the teenager manage this interaction to minimise his vulnerability?

NOTES FOR THE THERAPIST

This can be difficult to direct successfully since the character can be judged as either genuine, criminal or simply of unknown intent. The main emphasis with the group should be on choosing a conservative interpretation that is safe. The task for the therapist is again to make explicit the processes that typical adolescents exercise implicitly.

The purpose is not to resolve the honesty or criminality of the character making the offer of a Discman, but to explore the steps in reasoning required to respond to such characters safely. For example, a variety of responses which could prove difficult to refute include:

- *Blunt rebuff:* 'I don't need a Discman. My pizza is nearly ready. I have to go.'

- *Assertive polite:* 'I'd like a Discman, but I wouldn't buy anything not in a shop without getting it checked out first.'

- *Humorous rejection:* 'I don't usually buy my audio gear in the same place I buy my pizzas.'

- *Sensibly cautious:* 'What happens if it doesn't work? If you have a receipt from the shop then I might consider a deal. If anything went wrong, I could bring it back to the shop.'

The Discman scenario can be extended to cover a range of offers and requests which may not always be in the best interests of the AS adolescent; for example, offers of goods, requests for money, encouragement to act illegally, etc.

Session 12: Parent feedback and discussion

At this stage the adolescents will have spent five consecutive sessions together and altogether nine sessions in each other's company. The group should have gelled and be interacting with each other. If gelling has not occurred then a review of what has been done to date is urgently needed. However, in practice it should be obvious before now whether (a) the group has gelled and (b) if parents are supporting the practice of the principles and lessons outside the group setting. This is not the occasion to give parents individual reports on how their son or daughter is developing. A more private venue is suited to that task. Therefore, the focus of this session is on (b) not on (a).

Use this session to recapitulate the main points of the intervention – extracted from the first two parental sessions. Assuming the effects questionnaires have been completed regularly, their purpose can be restated briefly. The activities for this session include the recapitulating:

- the main goals of the intervention

- primary methods used

- parental role and commitment

- important pragmatic principles.

This is followed by feedback from the therapist about:

- general performance of the group

- improvements in specific areas of interaction

- behaviours that could be problematical

- satisfaction with parental input and support

- parent and adolescent social diary – compliance?

- areas where parental input requires attention.

Parents are invited by the therapist to give their feedback and questions:

- Are parents happy to continue?

- what difficulties have they faced with the social calendar?

- Have they changes in mind?

- Are any suggestions feasible within the intervention?

Session 13: Asking for help 1

At this stage, the intervention shifts emphasis away from an explicit didacticism and towards continuously evolving interactions and role plays.

SCENARIO FOR ROLE PLAY

A teenager has been given a new locker in his school. He is having trouble opening the locker. Students around him are filling their lockers and heading off to an important science class. The teenager becomes frustrated and does not ask for help. He continues fidgeting with the lock long after the others have gone to class. He attempts to bring his bag into the class but another student tells him that bags are banned. He becomes very upset.

How can he manage this problem temporarily and still attend class?

MODELLED SOLUTION

He still cannot open the locker, but now asks one of the students if he can share his locker until he sees a maintenance man after class. The other student agrees to this and both stride off to the class satisfied.

TOPICS

Intervention goal(s):

- Self-monitoring to aid setting priorities
- Shifting focus from detail to larger purpose
- Asking for help and negotiating

Social goals:

- Learning to use self-monitoring to cue asking for help

    Subgoals:

    - Responding to peer advice

    - Part-whole assessment

    - Identifying ineffective social behaviour

    - Using the social environment for support

NOTES FOR THE THERAPIST

Here the teenager is experiencing anxiety and possibly beginning to panic. When this occurs, clear thinking is no longer possible. The routine expectation of the AS teenager has been violated, leaving him confused and stressed. Before an alternative solution is realisable, the anxiety must be under control.

Session 14: Asking for help 2
SCENARIO FOR ROLE PLAY

A teenager is waiting for the school bus. He is in his school uniform. He is alone until another teenager, a stranger, arrives. The stranger is a boy of the same age wearing the same school uniform. The teenager does not attempt interaction with the stranger. The stranger looks around before initiating a conversation. The stranger requests the bus fare because he has lost his own. The stranger asks for the fare and struggles to get the teenager's attention. The teenager is brusque. The stranger becomes disheartened and leaves.

How can the teenager assess the stranger's request safely?

MODELLED SOLUTION

The teenager is more enquiring and tries to establish the grounds for trusting the stranger. He asks him about where he lives, why he has not met him before, etc. In the end he may choose to buy a ticket for the stranger (he does *not* give him money), or he may not.

NOTES FOR THE THERAPIST

The key distinction between the versions is the teenager's failure to read the distress of the stranger in his body language and facial expressions. Facial expressions, body language, eye gaze (reading the mind in the eyes) and tone of voice are very important here.

TOPICS

Intervention goals:

- Learning to respond to requests for help appropriately
- Assessing requests for help
- Learning to assess people
- Exploring alternative action routes
- Maintaining personal space

Social goals:

- Responding to strangers politely
- Assessing multiple points of contact
- Learning a safety strategy
- Learning to be assertive in countering requests for help

Subgoals:

- Learning to be assertive

- Evaluating others' reactions to behaviour

- Re-evaluating decisions

Session 15: Negotiation and compromise
SCENARIO FOR ROLE PLAY

A teenager is watching his favourite television programme. His cousin is staying in the house for a few days on vacation. Both are of similar age. The cousin comes into the room and takes the remote control. He points out that they agreed that he could watch his programme at this time and refuses to give back the remote control. The teenager wants to watch his programme. The teenager challenges his cousin's actions and stands in front of the television. He does not listen to his cousin's point of view. He explains that this is his favourite programme and since the cousin is in his house, he will just have to put up with it. He then reluctantly listens to his cousin's point of view but doesn't acknowledge that his cousin may have a valid point about the importance of keeping promises.

How could the teenager most effectively manage this dispute?

MODELLED SOLUTION

The teenager challenges his cousin's actions politely and asks him to explain himself. He actively listens to his cousin's point of view. He suggests to his cousin that a compromise be considered, otherwise the dispute will escalate and both of them may lose television time.

NOTES FOR THE THERAPIST

In the ineffective version, he has no interest in understanding his cousin's motivations or desires. His desire to watch the television is primary and any obstruction is dismissed as unreasonable. In the modelled solution, he listens to his cousin, presents his own case calmly and assertively, and acknowledges his cousin's point that he should keep his promise even if he does not want to. He apologises for dominating the television and ignoring his promise. He points out that his cousin's actions were unacceptable, but they should work out a compromise and put the issue behind them in the interests of building friendship. Facial expressions, eye contact, body language and tone of voice are very important here.

TOPICS

Intervention goals:

- Perspective taking as the basis for understanding others

- Reasonable commitments should be honoured

- Give and take is better than isolation

Social goals:

- Learning to negotiate and compromise

  Subgoals:

  - Explain viewpoint and offer justifications

  - Listen to responses

  - Acknowledge others' points of view

  - Identify own goal but be flexible and reasonable

  - Offer alternatives

  - Suggest referee/arbitration if in doubt

Session 16: Responding to criticism
SCENARIO FOR ROLE PLAY

A group of teenagers are sitting in a class. It is an unsupervised study period. One teenager keeps tapping his foot repetitively. The others find this mannerism very distracting. Eventually, they react. The teenager expresses no interest in being conciliatory and adjusting his manner. The group becomes angry.

How should the teenage respond sensibly to the criticism?

MODELLED SOLUTION

The teenager apologises for his mannerism, promises to control it and asks the others to remind him if he starts again.

NOTE FOR THE THERAPIST

The teenager accepts that his behaviour has been inconsiderate, apologises and promises to improve self-monitoring. Most importantly, he invites the group to help him monitor his behaviour and signal when he needs to adjust it.

TOPICS

Intervention goals:

- Responding to criticism

- Learning to self-monitor

- Considering others' perspectives

- Adjusting annoying behaviour is beneficial

- Learning to accept and respond to criticism

- Inviting others to cue behavioural adjustments

    Subgoals:

    - Taking responsibility for actions

    - Perspective on alienating behaviour

    - Apologising as a communication strategy

Session 17: Avoiding giving offence to others

SCENARIO FOR ROLE PLAY

> A school has closed early due to a heating problem. It is raining. A group of teenagers decides to shelter in the home of a classmate close by. Talk turns to sport. The others jibe a teenager in the group who is not a sports fan. The teenager has a tantrum when he cannot talk about himself and the others leave.

How could the teenager more effectively make his point and not sabotage the social gathering?

MODELLED SOLUTION

The teenager copes with the jibes and asks for turn taking and consideration from the others. The teenager participates assertively, sets boundaries around his interests, asks for turn taking in topics, and avoids emotive language.

NOTES FOR THE THERAPIST

The role play should emphasise the importance of using conversation to seek positive attention. People with AS often display negative cognitions and emotions in their interactions with others. These displays produce rejection responses in typical peers and it is important to coach those with AS to be consistently constructive. This is also why the banned phrases rule is so valuable.

TOPICS

Intervention goals:

- Monitoring agreement and disagreement in conversation
- Coping with being teased
- Learning to control emotions and relax
- Identifying strategies to preserve self-esteem
- Additional conversational strategies
- Seeking positive rather than negative attention
- Acknowledging others may have valid interests other than oneself

  Subgoals:

  - Avoid aggravating utterances and behaviour
  - Be politely assertive
  - Ask for turn taking
  - Topic management

Session 18: Managing anger
SCENARIO FOR ROLE PLAY

One teenager has agreed to bring takeaway meals over to another teenager's house so they can watch a movie. When he arrives, the other teenager rejects the meal and has a tantrum. The meal ends up on the floor and the teenager in a tantrum storms off to his room.

How can the teenager best manage his disappointment in the interests of friendship?

MODELLED SOLUTION

The teenager compromises and accepts the meal.

NOTES FOR THE THERAPIST

In the ineffective version, the teenager is in a rage. In the solution, he asserts that the meal is not to his liking but compromises in the interests of friendship. One compromise may involve him eating what he can of the meal. Another may involve his friend offering to share his meal to make up for the mistake – assuming two different meals. In any event, the emphasis is on coping with disappointment and realising that anger management is crucial to good social interactions and friendship maintenance.

TOPICS
Intervention goals:

- Frustration control

- Anger management

- Negotiation and compromise

- Dealing with unsatisfied desires

- Coping with disappointment

- Compromise for better future outcome

    Subgoals:

    - Self-monitoring and relaxation practice

    - Express disappointment politely

    - Avoid tantrum outbursts

    - Anger loses friends

Session 19: Common sense and impulse control
SCENARIO FOR ROLE PLAY

> A teenager has decided to tidy his room, and get rid of his old notebooks. He is discussing the task with a classmate at home. The teenager is not sure how best to go about the task. The classmate offers a number of suggestions, only to have all rejected. Finally, he concludes with a throwaway remark, '*You should throw them away.*' The teenager counters all the suggestions and opts for the extreme solution.

How should the teenager determine a sensible solution?

MODELLED SOLUTION

The teenager thanks the friend for listening to him talk about his predicament and apologises for boring him. He then asks the friend what he would do if he were at home in his house with the same predicament. The friend replies that he would pack the books in bags and ask his parents to take them to the recycling bin.

NOTE FOR THE THERAPIST

In the ineffective version, the teenager displays obsessional behaviour and is entirely self-absorbed. Decision making often gives rise to a predicament in AS. In the modelled solution, he imposes self-regulation and asks the friend to help him monitor his choices for common-sense outcomes.

TOPICS

Intervention goals:

- Learning to appraise consequences

- Assessing behaviour relative to others' behaviour

- Experimenting with embracing another's perspective

- Grasping consequences of literalism

- Impulse control

- Understanding the common-sense expectations of peers

  Subgoals:

  - Assess plan/goal for commonsense

  - Asking others to help monitor behaviour

  - Differentiating between likely outcome and intended outcome

Session 20: Parents and the real world

This is similar to the previous parental session.

TOPICS

- Logistics of organising social contact between the adolescents.

- Report on activities involving the adolescents in 'real world'.

- Parental inputs and expectations.

- Feedback from school and home.

- Evidence of carryover.

- Concerns and questions.

Session 21: Coping with bullying.
SCENARIO FOR ROLE PLAY

> A group of teenagers is sitting in a class. One teenager arrives back from holidays wearing a new jacket. Another teenager, the ringleader in the group, objects to the jacket and uses it as an excuse for harassment. The victim is not assertive but retreats into a passive response. The bully crows over him and stops when one of his henchmen reports the imminent arrival of a teacher.

What strategies are open to the teenager in these situations that offer the best outcome?

MODELLED SOLUTION

The victim refuses to be harassed and points out to the bully that he will report the matter to the teacher under the school's anti-bullying policy.

NOTES FOR THE THERAPIST

This session touches on the subject of bullying, something which all those with AS will have in common. There is no simple approach to dealing with bullying. It is important to emphasise that bullying behaviour is wrong. No one should be victimised. The victim is not at fault. The bully is to blame. The group should be encouraged to tell an adult if they are being bullied. In general, it is best to 'plug' any recommendations into a school's anti-bullying policies. The important things to note are that (a) the bullied child cannot be expected to deal with the matter without support; (b) all bullying needs to be addressed with urgency and a firm stop put to it; and (c) the cooperation of the school is vital to a satisfactory outcome.

TOPICS

Intervention goals:

- Responding to bullying
- Learning to be assertive
- Using school policy as part of strategy
- Learning to be appropriately assertive
- Use 'I' statements to express point of view

Subgoals:

- Assert what is mine
- Identify damaging/hurtful behaviour
- Look for support in the larger environment

Session 22: Setting boundaries and assessing risk

SCENARIO FOR ROLE PLAY

> A teenager is having a burger in a restaurant. Another group of teenagers sits down at the same table. Some of these are in his class in school. They immediately include him in conversation. They are laughing and giggling. He is very pleased with this. One of them produces a joint and passes it around. He is invited to take a few puffs. He takes the joint, smokes it publicly and attracts the manager's attention. The others flee as the manager holds on to him and rings the police.

How can the teenager safely manage such interactions with peers?

MODELLED SOLUTION

He is polite, but assertively declines to take the joint. He makes his excuses and leaves. This is a situation where stock responses may prove very helpful.

NOTES FOR THE THERAPIST

The presence of illicit drugs is ubiquitous and it is unlikely that the adolescent with AS can entirely avoid being presented with drug taking choices. The points to emphasise are that (a) drugs are illegal and breaking the law can have serious consequences; (b) drugs are inherently unhealthy for whole person develop-ment. How attracted are those with AS to illicit drugs? This is a difficult question to answer. On the positive side, most people with AS are very rule con-scious and tend to abide by the law. On the risk side, many adolescents with AS are socially excluded and in the right (or wrong) circumstances the company of a marginalised group of delinquents may be very attractive. In any event, the therapist should stress the illegal nature of drug taking and the career and health implications entailed.

TOPICS

Intervention goals:

- Analysing social situations

- Learning to read risky situations

- Developing self-protection strategies

- Resisting peer pressure

- Setting sensible boundaries

- Understanding and establishing social boundaries

- Assessing the interaction value against possible consequences

- Negotiating within a risky and tricky situation

    Subgoals:

    − Avoid aggravating utterances and behaviour

    − Using and not using emotive judgements

    − Declining politely

    − Learning social extraction strategies

Session 23: Friends − sharing experiences 1
SCENARIO FOR ROLE PLAY

A teenager drops in on another teenager for a snack and to show off several new graphic comics he has bought. The visitor fails to notice that his friend is upset and continues talking about the comics as if nothing is the matter. The upset friend reports that his sister has been in a road traffic accident and he is unsure if she will survive. He is waiting for his father to arrive home. The visiting friend wonders if there is any food in the house as he is hungry. The visitor carries on regardless of his friend's distress.

How should the visiting teenager conduct himself in these circumstances?

MODELLED SOLUTION

The visitor acknowledges that his friend is upset and asks if he can help in anyway.

NOTE FOR THE THERAPIST

In the solution, the visitor gives his friend room to *share* his information about his sister and *share* his distress. The expectations of the friend impose constraints on the range of behaviours appropriate to the visitor.

TOPICS

Intervention goals:

- Empathy and perspective taking
- Primacy of listening, rather than talking
- Expressing empathy – verbally and nonverbally
- Recognising distress in others
- Developing listening skills

   Subgoals:

   – In moments of distress think of the other person

   – Express sympathy politely

   – Avoid self-focus

   – Offer practical assistance

   – Active listening

Session 24: Friends – sharing experiences 2

SCENARIO FOR ROLE PLAY

The school debating champion is a girl. A teenage boy has taken an interest in her. He decides to ring her. In order to do so, he must obtain her number from his sister's mobile phone. He sneaks the number, without his sister knowing, and rings the girl without any subtlety. She is not interested in a date. The girl is surprised and tries to conclude the conversation politely.

How should the boy conduct such interactions while minimising the risk of offence to others?

MODELLED SOLUTION

He is polite, introduces himself, sets the context and asks her for a date. She is polite but declines and offers the promise of a chat after school in the future. He accepts her choice.

NOTE FOR THE THERAPIST

Sharing experiences is important to friendship and forming attachments to others. However, strategies for achieving desires do not always work out because the other person may not share the same desire. This is particularly the case in dating situations. One person may have something in common with another but that is not sufficient for the other person to agree to a date. This problem is frequently encountered by those with AS and can be traced back to their mind-reading difficulties.

TOPICS

Intervention goals:

- Learning to initiate conversation with the opposite sex

- Maintaining appropriate conversation on the phone

- Accepting that another's goal may be different

- Negotiation and listening in dating

- Perspective taking and learning to accept a 'no' for an answer

- Creating positive impressions with listeners

  Subgoals:

  – Desires are not always satisfiable

  – Tantrums are destructive

  – Foster long-term good relations

  – There is always tomorrow

Session 25: Adolescents – review and the future

This session should conclude on a high note. If possible, a nice meal together might be appropriate. The purpose of the session is to assess how far the intervention went in meeting the group's expectations. Recapitulate the aims and objectives of the intervention.

The therapist is in a position to identify strengths and areas that need further work. This includes the content and delivery of the intervention. It is a good time to identify what could be included in booster sessions in the future.

It is important to emphasise to the group that they stay in touch. Once they move out from under the umbrella of the intervention, the onus is largely with the parents. If at this stage some participants are not receiving 'good' school interaction reports, the reasons should be pursued. Possibly another type of intervention should be considered. However, it would be unusual for participants to remain with any intervention for this length of time and not exhibit some improvement.

The fundamental importance attaches neither to the intervention, nor to the therapist's investment in it, but to the progress being made by a participant. If progress is not being made, then a different approach may be required for that person. Interventions are now offered in so many modalities that participants should be encouraged to try other approaches if needs be.

Session 26: Parents – review and the future

This session marks both the end of one journey and the beginning of another. It is useful to run through the basic components of the intervention again, their role in it as coaches, their responsibilities to support interactions outside the group and their willingness to keep up contact with each other.

This is also the time to provide parents with any formal measures of feedback or to ask them to complete post-intervention questionnaires. Perhaps, most use can be made of this session by helping them plan a rota of social contact for the next three months. At the end of that time, they should return for a booster session.

Now is also the time to solicit comprehensive feedback from them and note suggestions they have for change. Any reservations, concerns or doubts they have about the coping skills of the adolescents should be addressed. Needless to add, but concluding on a constructive note is important.

Homework materials

Are written homework exercises worthwhile? Interventions and therapists differ on this issue. There is an argument that written homework improves comprehension of the sessions. However, there is no point in giving written homework to a group unless it will be corrected and returned. This will consume time outside the intervention and eat into time inside each session. A better approach is to ensure that participants contact each other between sessions. Even a phone text message is a start.

Conclusions

A good therapist will adapt whatever material is suitable to meet the needs of the participants. This is a fundamental aspect of best practice. What we have tried to do in this chapter is lay out a collection of criteria, mainly heuristic, to assist with making the most appropriate choices.

Locking into one methodology to the exclusion of others is probably unhelpful in addressing a heterogeneous condition like Asperger syndrome.

There are several lessons in the old story (Murphy 1999 includes a slightly different version) about a man who was out one night when he came across a colleague searching for something under a street light. He asked his colleague what was the matter. 'I have lost my wallet,' he replied. Well, the questioner thought, I'd better help out. After what seemed a long time searching to no avail, the questioner asked his colleague, 'Are you sure you lost your wallet?' He was sure and despite further searching neither man could find it. Perplexed, the questioner asked his colleague whether he could remember where he lost his wallet. 'Oh, over there, somewhere down the road,' he replied with eyes fixed on the ground.

'Then why on earth are you looking here?' asked the questioner.

'The light is brighter here. There's only a glimmer of light down there,' responded his colleague.

The lesson of this tale is that a solution is not always found where the light appears brightest. Often the solution may be less well illuminated, on roads less travelled. Therapists should try to engage with what works in terms of what meets the clients' expectations, rather than insist that the 'light' is okay but the client is in the dark.

9 Evaluation Issues

Now is a good time to read Chapter 1 again to remind yourself of your starting point and your expectations. The intervention aims to improve the quality and quantity of both neutral and enjoyable social interactions with peers, and to reduce the frequency of negative self-annihilating social interactions with peers. Over time, the therapist should notice that the group is becoming more relaxed. This can be done by direct observation of how they greet each other, the amount of conversation that occurs at break time, whether they are making contact with each other outside the group setting, self-reports of social contacts with peers (careful assessment needed) and parental reports of their social activities. Positive complimentary social interactions improve self-esteem and lay the foundations for adult relationships. How can we tell what is really happening?

Any evaluation must be matched to the aims of the intervention. This is an essential tenet. Objectives and their evaluation are interdependent. Our objectives have always been to effect modest improvements in social interaction with peers with accompanying improvements in self-esteem and self-confidence.

Evaluating the content and delivery of an intervention is a useful exercise. It helps identify strengths and weaknesses that will feed back into another iteration of the intervention. Regular progress reports from a variety of informants are useful. Pre-testing and post-testing of participants is leaning more towards the necessary and useful.

Appropriate post-intervention instruments are not abundant, particularly because of the wide variety of change variables up for measurement. We have found a combination of the Vineland, SDQ, our short social effects questionnaire and regular parent/school reports provide a level of confidence in post-intervention progress reports. The absence of a specific pragmatic communication instrument for post-testing is countered somewhat by examining recordings of conversations for evidence of improved prosody, decreased repetitions and PRS-related categories. The process is time consuming and the conversations reproduced in the relative security of the group may not occur outside. Concerns about data validity therefore arise. Perhaps the main questions that need to be addressed at a practical evaluation level are:

1. Did the group demonstrate the capacities and skills in interactions?

2. Is there evidence of carryover from third-party reports?

3. How reliable are the third-party reports?

The first bugbear infecting evaluation studies is that no two therapists are alike. Inevitably, the question arises: Who trains the therapists? Regrettably, it is a question without a simple reassuring answer. Occasionally there will be a hopefully healthy tension between recognising what needs addressing in a particular session (or with a particular participant) and who is best suited to the task. Demarcation disputes obviously should not spill into the group. Second, partitioning of skills and responsibilities is important both for the efficacy of the intervention and its evaluation. Without agreement in this area, any evaluation may end up 'pear-shaped' due to mismatch between intervention content and delivery and evaluation goals.

Evaluation is important

Judging the success of an intervention for AS adolescents is complex for a number of reasons. First, separating improvements due to the intervention from improvements due to developmental changes (or external circumstances) is difficult and ambiguous. Ideally, evidence of the transformation of strategies explored in the intervention into more qualitatively sophisticated rules is required.

Second, the generalisation of rules beyond the setting of the intervention is clearly desirable. However, collecting evidence of generalisation is nontrivial. It is impossible to conduct a dense sampling of social interactions and interpersonal/social problem-solving events that are representative of a person's demeanour over a reasonable period (several months). Third-party reports of generalisation are welcome – that generalisation occurred at all is marvellous.

Third, interventions for AS adolescents by their very nature give the AS adolescent extra attention. It is difficult to argue against the proposition that special treatment and lots of praise encourages more confidence and assertiveness. Bauminger (2002) in assessing her intervention specifically identifies 'special attention' as possibly having beneficial but difficult to measure side effects.

Fourth, in many cases it is likely that the group intervention is the first experience an AS adolescent has had of feeling safe with peers and enjoying being with peers. The group intervention emphasises that it is okay to be different. The participants can safely 'try out' having friends. The experience can help in shifting their self-concept. This is likely to increase social confidence and encourage the adolescents to be more open to new ways of thinking and behaving in social situations.

Again, successful role play in the group is likely to increase social confidence. These successes can prepare them for experimental interactions with peers outside of the group. A corollary is that often it is next to impossible to identify categorically which specific parts of an intervention have had specific and identifiable effects. The tendency, and it circumvents the question, is to see the combination of all the parts as the net contributor to any benefits – a holistic explanation.

Finally, while a range of assessment instruments exists for adolescents, none is likely to cover every feature of an intervention for AS adolescents. Consequently, therapists are pushed into using a variety of measures in an attempt to assess different effects. The extent to which the different measures are compatible is a moot point. The central effects that therapists (and other involved parties) need to note in AS adolescent interventions are:

- changes in social interaction styles and social behaviours – these should include frequency and quality improvements

- qualitative changes in speech production and conversation

- demonstration of nonverbal skills aligned to peer interactions

- observable changes in socio-emotional expression and reaction

- evidence of contingency management when confronted with interpersonal and social problems

- changes in self-regulation of emotions and behaviours.

It is preferable that these reports be garnered from other parties and not stop at therapists' impressions of improvements. The combination of parent and teacher observations can help identify any enhanced social performance of the AS adolescent. Peer reports may seem ideal but if they lead to furthering stigmatising of a participant careful consideration of their long-term effect is required.

If the participants are not interacting in a relaxed and interested manner with each other in the group setting, they will not interact in a relaxed fashion with typical peers. If the desired social interaction capacities are not demonstrated in the group setting then something is not working. Identifying this 'something' can be personally challenging to a therapist. The 'fault' may lie with the delivery of the materials, the management of the group, a lack of understanding of the social difficulties implied by AS, or a mismatched group. Let us be candid on this point: teaching social interaction skills to AS adolescents is not easy.

Lack of progress may also be due to an incomplete assessment of a participant. Interventions aimed at children and adolescents with behavioural difficulties without AS assume that the social skills they offer are learnable (Dowrick 1986). This assumption about the learnability of social skills needs considerable qualification and reinterpretation when addressing AS group interventions. For a start, the period for determining progress may be much longer than expected. Expectations that improvements in social interaction will occur on a par with expectations derived from similar interventions for non-AS groups will not stand.

Relying solely on the adolescents' reports alone for feedback is not adequate. For example, in questioning a participant about their social contacts in the previous week, he or she may reply that they met *someone, somewhere* in town, and did *a few things* together. The indefiniteness and vagueness of the reports tells us little if anything. Vague reports of social interactions should alert the therapist to probe the matter further with parents (or teachers, if the parents give permission). Again, the AS adolescent may be signalling either that he does not want to appear to be without friends or else is clumsily introducing a social bias that will be received well by the therapist.

Who to ask? Parental follow-up

The intervention demands that parents give up an amount of their time. However, a number of them may not be in a position to contribute as much of their time as the intervention demands. Some parents will have more to offer by way of time, resources and native understanding than others. If a parent does not bring their adolescent to a social outing, one can but encourage the parent to do better next time or else suggest a link-up with another parent for support. In the interests of promoting social interaction with peers outside the group, being firm with parents is as important as being firm with their offspring. Once the terms and conditions for participation are jointly understood and agreed, the therapist can rightly assert her expectations of parents.

Not sure if it is working: what to do?

Friendship as a means of self and other exploration, affiliation and identity construction is not usually grasped by those with AS. In our experience, it is widespread for AS adolescents to refer to friends and being in conversation with
friends, while parents and teachers report the contrary. In not all cases but in
many, friends are almost anyone who says hello or pays even slight attention to
the AS individual. The purpose behind double-checking reports of social interactions is to avoid premature evaluation of an intervention's success.

> Connor was a 16-year-old boy who had a diagnosis of AS since the age of
> ten. He had been bullied at school in every year. He frequently reported
> minor rule infringements by his peers to his teachers. Further eroding
> peer tolerance of his behaviour was his disparagement of their musical,
> reading and sporting interests. He left school at the age of 14 years. Three
> months before his sixteenth birthday, he was persuaded to participate in
> the social interaction intervention. He managed to relax and participate
> responsively after four sessions. However, his attachment to critical
> comment was carefully monitored and managed. Connor began having
> successful interactions in the group and sent phone texts to the other
> participants outside the group setting. He regained enough confidence to
> return to the school. This was an immensely brave step and his reports of
> interactions were of great interest. Despite frequently reporting that he
> had been talking and meeting with someone, somewhere and doing
> something, parental and school enquiries revealed that his social
> initiations in school were minimal. More often than not, he was invited
> into conversations. Connor's presentation of his successes reveals the
> unreliability of self-report and the absolute need to pursue and practise
> generalisation strategies.

We encourage feedback by way of an effects questionnaire that is distributed
on a regular basis to the parents (and teachers if parents ask) and after session
debriefings. We cautiously assess verbal reports from the adolescents about the
impact of the intervention.

> Evan is the father of a 15-year-old boy with AS. His son Thomas had been
> diagnosed at the age of eight years. In school, Thomas was provided with a
> classroom assistant to support his learning and prevent him being bullied.
> His parents had enrolled him in several groups over the years, and he
> attended social skills courses at least once a year. In their initial induction
> interview, Evan and his wife reported being 'disappointed' with the results
> of their previous efforts. They did not have 'high hopes' of yet another
> intervention. Over the following four to eight weeks, however, they

reported that Thomas seemed to enjoy the group and looked forward to each session. They also reported that he appeared much calmer and this was confirmed by his school. Most importantly, they mentioned that he had developed 'some type of friendship' with a classmate that led to regular outings to the cinema. Evan commented, when midway through the intervention, that he and a number of other parents were very sceptical at first that bringing 'all Aspergers together' would be effective. He was both surprised and pleased that the myth had been shaken. When speaking to Thomas about his interest in the group and what he might see in it to recommend to others, he replied promptly that he found 'it was great to be with others on the same road'. As a matter of record, all those that have been through the intervention have expressed exactly similar beliefs and feelings. For Thomas, like many others, the group was a place of acceptance and witness to his first sustainable social engagements. Over a period of months Thomas's confidence improved to the extent that he joined a sports club and began to learn volleyball skills. This was a big step forward in his social life.

Bernard was a 16-year-old boy with AS. He had come to the intervention having tried a number of other programmes. Bernard had a pronounced tendency to talk off topic. Most conversations would 'reduce' to monologues on his personal experiences and interpretations. During a session on friendship, he asked to leave the room as he was too upset. He did not have any friends in school and apart from exploitative acquaintances he had never had a friend. On the way home with his father that evening, he suddenly realised that for the first time in his life he had friends. He promptly began sending text messages to the other members of the group, thanking each for simply being there and being his friend.

Rosalind was a difficult oppositional 17-year-old girl according to her parents and teachers. She sat away from the rest of her classmates and referred to them in derogatory terms. On the surface, she simply did not 'get along with others'. Within three weeks of joining the intervention she made friends with another boy. In fact, they became sufficiently comfortable with each other for her to propose visiting him by train. In the weeks before this journey we had dealt with anxiety management, explaining that periods of anxiety will pass, and that repetition of this to oneself will help reduce the anxiety. The topics we focused upon were doing sports in school and managing unfamiliar tasks. Rosalind returned from her weekend trip very pleased. She told her mother that she was terrified of travelling alone by train but realised that the train journey time would end. Her mother replied that she thought it very brave to tackle such a task. It should be noted that this was Rosalind's first solo trip by train.

Ideally, these cases would be complemented by an extended evaluation over time. A rigorous evaluation using a control group excluded from the intervention is the ultimate evaluation model. However, interventions are not commonly available. Those that are accessible are often of short duration. There are also ethical concerns about excluding one needy group from an intervention in the absence of ready alternatives, which is why the use of third-party and self-reports is a reasonable best practice compromise.

At the end of the day, the success of the intervention depends to a large degree on the understanding, enthusiasm, humour and innovativeness of the therapists in collaboration with the group.

A small profit is better than none

People with Asperger syndrome often attribute aggression to processes and other people in their environment. Very often they feel persecuted. This has a basis in fact. Frequently peers increase the anxiety of the AS adolescent by misinterpreting their nonverbal behaviour. Unstable interpersonal relations, impulsivity and recurrent suicidal behaviour gestures are also prevalent. As noted in Chapter 7, a high rate of other psychiatric conditions is quite common among an Asperger syndrome group.

One cannot expect consistently to meet the needs of every adolescent with AS. The variety of life experiences and impairments is very wide within the autistic spectrum. One should aspire to doing *the most for the most*, and even that may not be enough. A lesson we have learnt about teaching interaction skills is that you can teach and practise all the strategies within the group setting, but some participants may still not enjoy putting these into operation with peers. Generalisation of skills, which entails the transference of learning to the external world, is hugely problematical for those with AS.

Conclusions

We have tried in this book to provide a range of methodological criteria for approaching interventions for adolescents with Asperger syndrome. Our approach is pluralistic and compatible with many therapies. The bulk of what has been outlined here can be imported and adapted to many therapies that have an emphasis on change through restructuring cognitions, behaviours and language skills. Accommodating the unidimensionality and the pared down psyche of the AS person are the main challenges for most therapies. However, unless psychoanalysis 'becomes' cognitive, it may be too difficult to fit the type of methods we outlined to it. People with Asperger syndrome are very concrete and literal in their thinking and complex psychoanalytic interpretations of the unconscious will probably confuse them – if not do more harm than good. Likewise, encounter group work that calls for aggressive confrontation with a person is incompatible with our suggestions.

Despite all the science and the hundreds of available therapies, we are still much better at suggesting what interventions should exclude rather than what they should include. There are good reasons for this hiatus. Developing and delivering an intervention for Asperger syndrome is a massive human re-engineering task. It is massive because of the scale of objective that must be met. It is a re-engineering task because the components have to be manufactured very publicly for the person with AS.

By way of analogy, diamonds come in two forms: natural and industrial. The natural diamond has been formed over eons through invisible processes in the earth. However, the industrial diamond must be explicitly engineered in much quicker time. On the one hand we have the result of natural 'evolutionary' processes, and on the other we have the result of applied understanding. Both will serve similar purposes though they have had different developmental histories. The process of industrial diamond production is analogous to the delivery of an intervention to those with Asperger syndrome. The challenge is to produce a similarly high quality result.

Adolescents with Asperger syndrome are fascinating, intriguing and sadly misunderstood young people. Fortunately, arising from their general loyalty to concrete thinking, facts and logic it will always be possible to move them forward based on truth.

APPENDIX I Relaxation Exercise

Clear your mind...

I'd like you to stand up now. [Pause.] Could you close your eyes while you listen to me? I'll tell you when to open them. Now I'd like you to take a few minutes to focus on the worries that you've brought here with you this evening.

There may be any number of things on your mind: whether you remembered to close your bedroom door [pause], put your favourite hobby items away [pause], perhaps things you left undone at home [pause], or things that you need to do tomorrow.

Take a minute to really focus on what those worries are for you right now [pause], and make a list in your head.

These concerns on your list are using your energy. They are stopping you from being fully present here this evening.

Probably there is nothing you can do during the next two hours about these worries, except to worry [pause], and that will distract you from all that you could be learning here [pause], so let's put these worries away for awhile.

I'd like you to create in your mind a big schoolbag [pause], and a lock and key [pause], but it needs to be large enough and strong enough to hold all the concerns on your list. [Pause.] Take a moment to visualise this bag as best you can. The bag is now in front of you, open.

Now, I'd like you to put each of your worries into the bag, one by one. [Pause.] Make sure they all go in. [Pause.] As they are going in say to yourself: There is nothing that I can do about this now [pause], so I am going to put these worries away in this safe, secure bag while I am here [pause], and I know that I can come back later and reclaim all of my concerns.

Now when you have put your worries and concerns in this bag, I'd like you to zip it up and lock it with your key. [Pause.] Now I'd like you to put the key away somewhere safe and remember that at the end of the session you can open the lock, unzip your bag and pick up where you left off.

And when you are ready, I'd like you to open your eyes and concentrate on what is happening here.

APPENDIX 2 Banned Phrases Sheet

Certain phrases are more likely to destroy our efforts than other phrases. They are the kind of phrases that destroy conversation. It is best to avoid these phrases until you know someone for a few months and only then use them *very* rarely. *The rules of this exercise are simple:*

1. Everyone participates
2. No one judges anyone else
3. Quantity is better than quality

Now try to list at least five phrases that could destroy a social learning group like ours.

1. I don't have the time for this.
2. This is ridiculous.
3. I did all right before this group.
4. Why should I change? I'm okay!
5. I'm not ready for this.
6. I've never done this before.
7. That's not my problem, it's yours.
8. It's not practical.
9. I've tried this before. It didn't work.
10. It just won't work, I know that.
11.
12.
13.
14.
15.

Action Plan Sheet

If you hear any good ideas or ways of doing something differently and better during a session or outside in the world, this is where you should write them down. If good ideas are not tried within a day, they are often forgotten.

When you get home, put this sheet in an important place in your bedroom where you can see it. Check every week how many of the good ideas you get to try out.

1. Pay more attention to my classmates.

2. Know about popular movies, music and sport.

3. Practise using stock phrases.

4. Interact for short periods.

5. Don't talk too long about my hobbies.

6.

7.

8.

9.

10.

11.

12.

13.

14.

APPENDIX 4 Getting Everyone to Interact Game

Guess Who?

Guess Who? is an easy game to play with a group of people. You don't need any materials. This is how it is played with the adolescents:

1. One person thinks of a famous person.

2. The others try to guess that famous person.

3. They can only ask questions with yes or no as an answer, for example:

    - *wrong*: Is the person a man or a woman?

    - *right*: Is the person a man?

    - *wrong*: Is he or she a scientist or a musician?

    - *right*: Is he or she a scientist?

4. Everybody takes turns in asking questions.

5. Only one question per turn is allowed.

Remember: encourage everyone to listen carefully to each other's questions and the answers, as it will help each to guess the correct answer sooner. Have fun!

Appendix 5 Charades – Ideal for AS Role Plays

Charades is a well-established group game. One person tries to describe a movie, book or television series using nonverbal communication solely. This involves gesturing and pointing when someone makes a 'good' guess. The person being quizzed, the 'performer', begins by identifying whether his or her topic is a movie (make the motion of a movie camera being wound by hand), a book (open out hands palm upwards as if supporting a book) or a television piece (draw a rectangular frame with fingers). Next, he or she shows by counting their fingers how many words are in the title. The group should signal that they comprehend his message ('So it's a movie, with five words in the title'). The performer should acknowledge responses and clearly signal if the responses are correct or incorrect. He or she may then attempt to convey the sounds of some words (or a word) in the title by (a) pulling at their ear ('sounds like' signal) and (b) following with a gesture related to the sound/word he or she wants to convey. Each person in turn, tries to guess the sound and the word. After several attempts the title will be either identified or else the performer will have 'won' and can then reveal the title. There are variations on charades but the emphasis on nonverbal communication in order to effect purposeful communication makes it ideal for AS children and adolescents.

A Sample Script

Here we present an example of a typical video script – it has been edited to save space. In the first version, an ineffective social script is enacted. The second version enacts an effective social script. As can be seen, the effective script illustrates a great number of pragmatic skills that are very banal, very commonplace but essential to effective social interaction. The choice of library assistant title is deliberate. The group is told that library assistants are students who work part time in the school (or college) library. This provides a justification for a peer assistant and student being of similar age. In practice this is the first video scenario we use to assess individual group member's comprehension of tone of voice, body language and perspective-taking skills (the assistant is performing mechanical tasks, rather than explicit mentalising tasks).

Library Scenario 1: Indicates lack of perspective taking. Adolescent does not recognise the assistant's preoccupation. Failure to ask for help appropriately (initiation deficit).

Opening shot from inside library shows adolescent entering the library and striding towards a particular shelf of books. It would be useful to have book categories on the shelves. Adolescent is seen browsing the shelf in an over-shoulder shot. He flicks through the spines of the books using his index finger. He conducts three searches to indicate thoroughness. He glances up at the main library desk after each scan of the shelf. He appears slightly perplexed, even annoyed. Finally, he approaches the desk. The library assistant is busy sorting some papers. Her body is slightly turned away from the desk. [*Important to get both parties in same camera shot.*]

Adolescent: I can't find the *Student Guide to the Internet*. Where is it?

Adolescent is leaning against desk and slightly forward. Speaks in a slightly raised monotone voice. Brusque. No eye contact. Looking past assistant.

Assistant: I don't think it is there.

Briefly, checks trolley beside her for book. Assistant glances up from work but otherwise appears unresponsive. Neutral tone.

Adolescent: Aaahh!

Adolescent sighs loudly and leaves without waiting for any reaction. Assistant glances up slightly puzzled as he leaves through door.

Library Scenario 2: Indicates perspective taking. Adolescent recognises the assistant's preoccupation. Makes eye contact. Initiates request for help appropriately. Speaks assertively but calmly. Observes, waits and listens during the interaction.

Opening shot from inside library shows adolescent entering the library and striding towards a particular shelf of books. It would be useful to have book categories on the shelves. User is seen browsing the shelf in an over-shoulder shot. User flicks through the spines of the books using his index finger. He conducts three searches to indicate thoroughness. He glances up at the main library desk after each scan of the shelf. He appears slightly perplexed, even annoyed. Finally, he approaches the desk. The assistant is busy sorting some papers. Her body is slightly turned away from the desk. [*Important to get both parties in same camera shot.*]

Adolescent: Hello. When you are ready please?

Adolescent is in front of desk and looking directly at the assistant. Waits a moment to study her actions. Speaks in a calm tone. Waits until the assistant looks up.

Assistant: Yes?

Assistant glances up from work but otherwise appears unresponsive. Speaks with a slight impatience.

Adolescent: When you are ready could you help me please?

Adolescent waits to establish eye contact. Calm polite tone.

Assistant: Right. How can I help you?

Assistant puts aside papers and looks directly at adolescent. She speaks in polite tone.

Adolescent: I am looking for the *Student Guide to the Internet* but it is not on the shelf.

Adolescent retains eye contact (doesn't stare) and position. Speaks calmly.

Assistant: It mustn't be there then. It is probably out on loan. I'll check the computer...No, it was returned this morning.

Assistant answers politely and taps away at a keyboard. Looks at adolescent when replying.

Adolescent: Could you check the book returns for it please? I need it for my school project.

Adolescent still speaks calmly and focuses on retaining eye contact.

Assistant: Fine. I'll look now. … Sorry it is not there but this note says that the book is having its cover glued back on this afternoon.

Assistant puts papers aside, looks up, nods an acknowledgment and speaks less formally. She turns around to check the returns trolley. Turns back with a piece of yellow paper in her hand.

Adolescent: Can I reserve it when it comes back?

Adolescent speaks calmly and uses an open face expression now that he has obtained the assistant's attention and cooperation.

Assistant: It should be possible. Give me your library card and I'll enter the details in the computer… Come back tomorrow afternoon and I'll have it reserved for you.

Assistant is more cooperative in tone. Reaches out for library card, and punches some keys. She hands back the card with a warmer expression on her face.

Adolescent: Thanks. I won't be able to return tomorrow afternoon, but I will return the day after to collect it, if that's okay. You have been very helpful.

The adolescent returns the card to his pocket. He nods with an open expression on his face.

Assistant: No problem. I'll reserve the book for the day after tomorrow. Sorry if I appeared preoccupied earlier, but the two other assistants are out sick today.

Assistant gives a friendly shrug of her shoulders and the adolescent waves a brief goodbye before exiting.

APPENDIX 7 Social Effects Questionnaire

Sample Social Effects Questionnaire: Social Interaction Therapy

Name: Parent: Date:

1 = no not at all, 2 = somewhat, 3 = more than twice, 4 = yes very much,
5 = done earlier

1.	Did your child talk about the intervention?	1	2	3	4
2.	Did your child talk about 'banned phrases'?	1	2	3	4
3.	Did your child talk about the relaxation exercises?	1	2	3	4
4.	Did your child talk about conversation skills?	1	2	3	4
5.	Did your child practise the relaxation exercises?	1	2	3	4
6.	Did you notice an improvement in conversation skills in your child?	1	2	3	4
7.	Did you notice an improvement in listening skills in your child?	1	2	3	4
8.	Did you notice a reduction of stress in your child?	1	2	3	4
9.	Did your child seek out topics that would be of common interest with his or her peers, e.g. sport, music?	1	2	3	4
10.	Did your child enjoy the intervention?	1	2	3	4

11.	Did you notice anything else in your child that could be related to the social skills training?					
12.	Are you helping your child to practise the recommendations of the programme?	1	2	3	4	
13.	If so how, and if not why not?					
14.	Recorded by you: frequency of peer interaction in last week	1	2	3	4	
15.	Recorded by you: quality of peer interactions (a) moderate but negative; (b) moderate but neutral; (c) moderate but improving					
16.	Were peer interactions: (a) worse than in past month; (b) same as last month; (c) an improvement on last month?					
17.	Recorded by school: frequency of peer interaction in last week	1	2	3	4	
18.	Recorded by school: quality of peer interactions (a) moderate but negative; (b) moderate but neutral; (c) moderate but improving					

References

Adams, C. (2002) 'Practitioner review: The assessment of language pragmatics.' *Journal of Child Psychology and Psychiatry 43*, 973–987.

Adams, C., Green, J., Gilchrist, A. and Cox, A. (2002) 'Conversational behaviour of children with Asperger syndrome and conduct disorder.' *Journal of Child Psychology and Psychiatry 43*, 679–690.

Adolphs, R., Sears, L.L. and Piven, J. (2001) 'Abnormal processing of social information from faces in autism.' *Journal of Cognitive Neuroscience 13*, 232–240.

Aijmer, K. (1996) *Conversational Routines in English: Convention and Creativity.* London: Addison Wesley Longman.

American Psychiatric Association (1994) *Diagnostic and Statistical Manual of Mental Disorders IV. Washington, DC: APA.*

Andersen-Wood, L. and Smith, B.R. (1997) *Working with Pragmatics.* Bicester: Speechmark.

Asher, N. and Lascarides, A. (2003) *Logics of Conversation.* Cambridge: Cambridge University Press.

Ashton, K. and Harpur, J. (2004) 'Critique of the PRS.' Maynooth, Computer Science Department, National University of Ireland Maynooth.

Asperger, H. (1944) 'Die autistischen psychopathen im kindesalter.' *Archiv fur Psychiatrie und Nervenkrankheiten 117*, 76–136.

Attwood, T. (1998) *Asperger's Syndrome: A Guide for Parents and Professionals. London: Jessica Kingsley Publishers.*

Attwood, T. (2000) 'Strategies for improving the social integration of children with Asperger syndrome.' *Autism 4*, 85–100.

Baltaxe, C. (1977) 'Pragmatic deficits in the language of autistic adolescents.' *Journal of Paediatric Psychology 2*, 176–180.

Bara, B.G., Bosco, F. M. and Bucciarelli, M. (1999) 'Developmental pragmatics in normal and abnormal children.' *Brain and Language 68*, 507–528.

Bara, B.G., Bucciarelli, M. and Colle, L. (2001) 'Communicative abilities in autism: evidence for attentional deficits.' *Brain and Language 77*, 216–240.

Baron-Cohen, S. (1988) 'Social and pragmatic deficits in autism: Cognitive or affective?' *Journal of Autism and Developmental Disorders 18*, 379–402.

Baron-Cohen, S. (1995) *Mindblindness: An Essay on Autism and Theory of Mind.* Cambridge MA: MIT Press.

Baron-Cohen, S. (2003) *The Essential Difference: Men, Women and the Extreme Male Brain.* Harmondsworth: Penguin.

Baron-Cohen, S. (2004) 'Autism: Research into causes and intervention.' *Pediatric Rehabilitation 7*, 73–78.

Baron-Cohen, S. and Swettenham, J. (1997) 'Theory of mind in autism: Its relationship to executive function and central coherence.' In D.J. Cohen, and F.R. Volkmar (eds) *Handbook of Autism and Pervasive Developmental Disorders.* New York: Wiley, pp.880–893.

Baron-Cohen, S., Ring, H.A., Bullmore, E.T., Wheelwright, S., Ashwin, C. and Williams, S.C.R. (2000) 'The amygdala theory of autism.' *Neuroscience & Biobehavioral Reviews 24*, 355–364.

Baron-Cohen, S., Wheelwright, S., Hill, J., Raste, Y. and Plumb, I. (2001) 'The "Reading the Mind in the Eyes" test revised version: A study with normal adults or adults with Asperger syndrome or high-functioning autism.' *Journal of Child Psychology and Psychiatry 42*, 241–252.

Barry, T.D., Klinger, L.G., Lee, J.M., Palardy, N., Gilmorr, T. and Bodin, S.D. (2003) 'Examining the effectiveness of an outpatient clinic-based social skills group for high-functioning children with autism.' *Journal of Autism and Development Disorders 33*, 685–701.

Barton, J.J.S., Cherkasova, M.V., Hefter, R., Cox, T.A., O'Connor, M. and Manoach, D.S. (2004) 'Are patients with social developmental disorders prosopagnosic? Perceptual heterogeneity in the Asperger and socio-emotional processing disorders.' *Brain: A Journal of Neurology 127*, 1706–1716.

Bartsch, K. and Wellman, H.M. (1995) *Children Talk About the Mind.* New York: Oxford University Press.

Bauman, M.L. and Kemper, T.L. (eds) (1994) *The Neurobiology of Autism.* Baltimore: Johns Hopkins University Press.

Bauminger, N. (2002) 'The faciliatation of social emotional understanding and social interaction in high-functioning children with autism: Intervention outcomes.' *Journal of Autism and Development Disorders 32*, 283–298.

Bauminger, N. and Kasarl, C. (1999) 'Brief report: Theroy of mind in high-functioning children with autism.' *Journal of Autism and Developmental Disorders 29*, 81–86.

Bettleheim, B. (1967) *The Empty Fortress: Infantiles, Autism and the Birth of the Self.* New York: Free Press.

Bishop, D.V.M. (1997) *Uncommon Understanding: Development and Disorders of Language Comprehension in Children.* Hove: Psychology Press.

Bishop, D.V.M. (1998) 'Development of the children's communication checklist (CCC): A method for assessing qualitative aspects of communicative impairment in children.' *Journal of Child Psychology and Psychiatry 39*, 379–402.

Bishop, D.V.M. (2003) *Children's Communication Checklist (CCC).* San Antonio, TX: Harcourt Assessment Inc.

Bishop, D.V.M. and Norbury, C.F. (2002) 'Exploring the borderlands of autistic disorder and specific language impairment: a study using standardised diagnostic instruments.' *Journal of Child Psychology and Psychiatry 43*, 917–929.

Bishop, D.V.M., Chan, J., Adams, C., Hartley, J. and Weir, F. (2000) 'Conversational responsiveness in specific language impairment: Evidence of disproportionate pragmatic difficulties in a subset of children.' *Journal of Development and Psychopathology 12*, 177–199.

Bjorn, K., Gillberg, C. and Hagberg, B. (1999) 'Brief report: Autism and Asperger syndrome in seven year old children: A total population survey.' *Journal of Autism and Developmental Disorders 29*, 327–331.

Blacher, J., Kraemer, B., Schalow, M., Ziatas, K., Durkin, K. and Pratt, C. (2003) 'Asperger syndrome and high functioning autism: Research concerns and emerging foci: Differences in assertive speech acts produced by children with autism, Asperger syndrome, specific language impairment, and normal development.' *Current Opinion in Psychiatry 16*, 535–542.

Blakemore, D. (2002) *Relevance and Linguistic Meaning: The Semantics and Pragmatics of Discourse Markers.* Cambridge: Cambridge University Press.

Bledsoe, R., Smith, B., and Simpson, R.L. (2003) 'Use of a social story intervention to improve mealtime skills of an adolescent with Asperger syndrome.' *Autism 7*, 289–295.

Bock, M.A. (2001) 'SODA strategy: Enhancing the social interaction skills of youngsters with Asperger syndrome.' *Intervention in School and Clinic 36*, 272–278.

Botvin, G.J. (2000) 'Preventing drug abuse in schools: Social and competence enhancement approaches targeting individual-level etiologic factors.' *Addictive Behaviors 25*, 887–897.

Boucher, J., Lewis, V. and Collis, G. (1998) 'Familiar face and voice matching and recognition in children with autism.' *Journal of Child Psychology and Psychiatry 39*, 171–181.

Bowler, D.M. (1992) '"Theory of mind" in Asperger syndrome.' *Journal of Child Psychology and Psychiatry 33*, 877–893.

Busceaum, J., Smith, C., Fitzgerald, M. and Davis, K. (1999) 'A genome wide linkage study in Autism.' *Molecular Psychiatry 41*, 73.

Cahill, L., McGaugh, M.L. and Weinberger, N.M. (2001) 'The neurobiology of learning and memory: Some reminders to remember.' *Trends in Neuroscience 24*, 578–581.

Camp, B.W., and Bash, M.A. (1981) *Think Aloud*. Champaign, IL: Research Press.

Carrington, S. and Graham, L. (2001) 'Perceptions of school by two teenage boys with Asperger syndrome and their mothers: A qualitative study.' *Autism 5*, 37–48.

Carruthers, P. (1996) 'Autism as mindblindness: An elaboration and partial defence.' In P. Carruthers and P.K. Smith (eds) *Theories of Mind*. Cambridge: Cambridge University Press, pp.257–273.

Carver, L. and Dawson, G. (2002) 'Development and neural bases of face recognition in autism.' *Molecular Psychiatry 7*, S18–S20.

Cederlund, M. and Gillberg, C. (2004) 'One hundred males with Asperger syndrome: A clinical study of background and associated factors.' *Developmental Medicine and Child Neurology 46*, 652–660.

Celani, G., Battacchi, M.W. and Arcidiacono, L. (1999) 'The understanding of the emotional meaning of facial expressions in people with Autism.' *Journal of Autism and Developmental Disorders 29*, 57–66.

Charman, T. (1999) 'Autism and pervasive developmental disorders.' *Current Opinions in Neurology 12*, 155–159.

Church, C., Alisanski, S. and Amanuallah, S. (2000) 'The social, behavioural and academic experiences of children with Asperger syndrome.' *Focus on Autism and Other Developmental Disabilities 15*, 12–21.

Constantino, J.N., Gruber, C.P., Davis, S., Hayes, S., Passanante, N. and Przybeck, T. (2004) 'The factor structure of autistic traits.' *Journal of Child Psychology and Psychiatry 45*, 719–726.

Cook, K.T. (2002) 'An analysis of two approaches to social skills instruction for students with Asperger syndrome.' Dissertation Thesis, University of Kansas.

Crick, F. (1995) *The Astonishing Hypothesis*. London: Touchstone.

Critchley, H.D., Daly, E.M., Bullmore, E.T., Williams, S.C., van Amelsvoort, T., Robertson, D.M., Rowe, A.M.P., McAlonan, G., Howlin, P. and Murphy, D.G. (2000) 'The functional neuroanatomy of social behaviour: Changes in cerebral blood flow when people with autistic disorder process facial expression.' *Brain 123*, 2203–2212.

Dahlgren, S.O. and Trillingsgaard, A. (1996) 'Theory of mind in non-retarded children with autism and Asperger syndrome: A research note.' *Journal of Child Psychology and Psychiatry 37*, 759–763.

Dennett, D. (1978) 'Beliefs about beliefs.' *Behavioural and Brain Sciences 4*, 568–570.

Dobbinson, S., Perkins, M.R. and Boucher, J. (1998) 'Structural patterns in conversations with a woman who has autism.' *Journal of Communication Disorders 31*, 113–134.

Dorris, L., Espie, C.A.E., Knott, F. and Salt, J. (2004) 'Mind-reading difficulties in the siblings of people with Asperger's syndrome: Evidence for a genetic influence in the abnormal development of a specific cognitive domain.' *Journal of Child Psychology and Psychiatry, and Allied Disciplines 45*, 412–418.

Dowrick, P.W. (1986) *Social Survival for Children: A Trainer's Resource Book*. New York: Brunner/Mazel.

Dowrick, P.W. (1999) 'A review of self modeling and related interventions.' *Applied and Preventive Psychology 8*, 23–39.

Edelman, G.M. (1994) *Bright Air, Brilliant Fire – On the Matter of the Mind*. Harmondsworth: Penguin.

Eggins, S. and Slade, D. (1997) *Analysing Casual Conversation*. London: Continuum Press.

Engstrom, I., Engstrom, L. and Emilsson, B. (2003) 'Psychosocial functioning in a group of Swedish adults with Asperger syndrome or high-functioning autism?' *Autism 7*, 99–110.

Etkin, A., Klemenhagen, K.C., Dudman, J.T., Rogan, M.T., Hen, R., Kandel, E.R. and Hirsch, J. (2004) 'Individual differences in trait anxiety predict the response of the basolateral amygdala to unconsciously processed fearful faces.' *Neuron 44*, 1043–1055.

Fallgatter, A.J., Ehlis, A.-C., Rosler, M., Strik, W.K., Blocher, D. and Herrmann, M.J. (2005) 'Diminished prefrontal brain function in adults with psychopathology in childhood related to attention deficit hyperactivity disorder.' *Psychiatry Research: Neuroimaging 138*, 157–169.

Fitzgerald, M. (2004) *Autism and Creativity.* London: Brunner-Routledge.

Fletcher, P.C., Happé, F., Frith, U., Baker, S.C., Dolan, R.J., Frackowiak, R.S.J. and Frith, C.D. (1995) 'Other minds in the brain: A functional imaging study of "theory of mind" in story comprehension.' *Cognition 57*, 109–128.

Fox, C.L. and Boulton, M.J. (2003) 'Evaluating the effectiveness of a social skills training (SST) programme for victims of bullying.' *Educational Research 45*, 231–247.

Foxx, R.M., McMorrow, M.J., Bittle, R.G. and Fenlon, S.J. (1985) 'Teaching social skills to psychiatric inpatients.' *Behaviour Research and Therapy 23*, 531–537.

Frankel, F., Cantwell, D.P. and Myatt, R. (1996) 'Helping ostracized children: Social skills training and parent support for socially rejected children.' In E.D.H.P.S. Jensen (ed) *Psychosocial Treatments for Child and Adolescent Disorders: Empirically Based Strategies for Clinical Practice.* Washington, DC: American Psychological Association, pp.595–617.

Frankel, F., Myatt, R., Cantwell, D.P. and Feinberg, D.T. (1997) 'Parent assisted transfer of social skills training: Effects on children with and without attention deficit hyperactivity disorder.' *Journal of the American Academy of Child and Adolescent Psychiatry 36*, 1056–1064.

Frith, U. (1989) 'A new look at language and communication in autism.' *British Journal of Disorders of Communication 24*, 123–150.

Frith, U. (2003) *Autism: Explaining the Enigma,* 2nd edn. Oxford: Blackwell Publishing.

Frith, U. (2004b) 'Emanuel Miller lecture: Confusions and controversies about Asperger syndrome.' *Journal of Child Psychology and Psychiatry 45*, 672–686.

Frith, U. and Happé, F. (1994) 'Autism: Beyond "theory of mind".' *Cognition 50*, 115–132.

Frith, U. and Houston, R. (2000) *Autism and History.* Oxford: Blackwell.

Gerland, G. (1997) *A Real Person: Life on the Outside.* London: Souvenir Press.

Ghaziuddin, M. (2005) *Mental Health Aspects of Autism and Asperger Syndrome.* London: Jessica Kingsley Publishers.

Gilchrist, A., Green, J., Cox, A., Burton, D., Rutter, M. and Le Courteur, A. (2001) 'Development and current functioning in adolescents with Asperger syndrome: A comparative study.' *Journal of Child Psychology and Psychiatry 42*, 227–240.

Gillberg, C. (2002) *A Guide to Asperger Syndrome.* Cambridge: Cambridge University Press.

Gillberg, C. and Coleman, M. (2000) *The Biology of the Autistic Syndromes.* Cambridge: MacKeith Press.

Goffman, E. (1971) *Relations in Public.* Harmondsworth: Penguin.

Goffman, E. (1981) *Forms of Talk.* Philadelphia: University of Pennsylvania Press.

Goffman, E. (1982) *Interaction Ritual,* 1st edn. London: Pantheon Books.

Goodman, R. (1999) 'The extended version of the Strengths and Difficulties Questionnaire as a guide to child psychiatric caseness and consequent burden.' *Journal of Child Psychology and Psychiatry 40*, 791–801.

Gopnik, A. and Meltzoff, A.N. (1998) *Words, Thoughts and Theories.* Cambridge, MA: MIT Press.

Grandin, T. (1996) *Thinking in Pictures and Other Reports from My Life with Autism.* New York: Vintage Books.

Grandin, T. and Scariano, M. (1986) *Emergence: Labeled Autistic.* New York: Warner Books.

Gray, C. (1994) *The Original Social Stories Book.* Austin, TX: Future Horizons.

Green, G. and Morgan, J. (1981) 'Pragmatics, grammar, and discourse.' In P. Cole (ed) *Radical Pragmatics.* New York: Academic Press.

Greenway, C. (2000) 'Autism and Asperger syndrome: Strategies to promote prosocial behaviours.' *Educational Psychology in Practice 16*, 469–486.

Grice, P. (1975) 'Logic and conversation.' In P. Cole and J.L. Morgan (eds) *Syntax and Semantics, Vol. 3: Speech Acts*. New York: Academic Press, pp.41–58.

Grice, P. (1989) *Studies in the Way of Words*. Cambridge, MA: Harvard University Press.

Grossman, J.B., Klin, A., Carter, A. and Volkmar, F.R. (2000) 'Verbal bias in recognition of facial emotions in children with Asperger syndrome.' *Journal of Child Psychology and Psychiatry 41*, 369–379.

Hadjikhani, N., Joseph, R.M., Snyder, J., Chabris, C.F., Clark, J., Steele, S., McGrath, L., Vangel, M., Aharon, I. and Feczko, E. (2004) 'Activation of the fusiform gyrus when individuals with autism spectrum disorder view faces.' *NeuroImage 22*, 1141–1150.

Hadwin, J., Baron-Cohen, S., Howlin, P. and Hill, K. (1997) 'Does teaching theory of mind have an effect on the ability to develop conversation in children with autism?' *Journal of Autism and Development Disorders 27*, 519–535.

Hampe, B. (1997) *Making Documentary Films and Reality Videos*. New York: Henry Holt.

Hanko, G. (1999) *Increasing Competence through Collaborative Problem-Solving*. London: David Fulton Publishers.

Happé, F.G.E. (1993) 'Communicative competence and theory of mind in autism: A test of relevance theory.' *Cognition 48*, 101–119.

Happé, F. (1999) 'Autism: Cognitive deficit or cognitive style?' *Trends in Cognitive Sciences 3*, 216–222.

Harpur, J., Bengtsson, L. and Lawlor, M. (2005) 'Maladaptive discourse constraints: Evidence for excessive coordiantion and subordination in conversations with Asperger syndrome subjects.' Paper presented at the conference 'Constraints in Discourse', Dortmund, Universität Dortmund.

Harpur, J., Lawlor, M. and Fitzgerald, M. (2003) *Succeeding in College with Asperger Syndrome: A Student Guide*. London: Jessica Kingsley Publishers.

Hatton, C. (1998) 'Pragmatic language skills in people with intellectual disabilities: A review.' *Journal of Intellectual and Development Disability 23*, 79–100.

Hill, E.L. (2004) 'Evaluating the theory of executive dysfunction in autism.' *Developmental Review 24*, 189–233.

Hill, E., Berthoz, S. and Frith, U. (2004) 'Brief report: Cognitive processing of own emotions in individuals with autism spectrum disorder and their relatives.' *Journal of Autism and Development Disorders 34*, 229–235.

Hobson, P. (1995) *Autism and the Development of Mind*. Hove: Psychology Press.

Hobson, P. (2002) *The Cradle of Thought: Challenging the Origins of Thinking*. London: Macmillan.

Holliday Willey, L. (1999) *Pretending to be Normal: Living with Asperger's Syndrome*. London: Jessica Kingsley Publishers.

Howlin, P. (1998) *Children with Autism and Asperger Syndrome: A Guide for Practitioners and Carers*. Chichester: Wiley.

Howlin, P. (2003) 'Outcome in high-functioning adults with and without early language delays: Implications for the differentiation between autism and Asperger syndrome.' *Journal of Autism and Development Disorders 33*, 3–13.

Howlin, P., Goode, S., Hutton, J. and Rutter, M. (2004) 'Adult outcome for children with autism.' *Journal of Child Psychology and Psychiatry 45*, 212–229.

Jackson, L. (2002) *Freaks, Geeks and Asperger Syndrome: A User Guide to Adolescence*. London: Jessica Kingsley Publishers.

Jolliffe, T. and Baron-Cohen, S. (1999) 'The strange stories test: A replication with high functioning adults with autism or Asperger syndrome.' *Journal of Autism and Developmental Disorders 29*, 395–406.

Jolliffe, T. and Baron-Cohen, S. (2001) 'A test of central coherence theory: Can adults with high-functioning autism or Asperger syndrome integrate fragments of an object?' *Cognitive Neuropsychiatry 6*, 193–216.

Kaland, N., Meller-Nielsen, A., Callesen, K., Mortensen, E.L., Gottlieb, D. and Smith, L. (2002) 'A new "advanced" test of theory of mind: Evidence from children and adolescents with Asperger syndrome.' *Journal of Child Psychology and Psychiatry 43*, 517–528.

Kanner, L. (1949) 'Problems of nosology and psychodynamics of early infantile autism.' *American Journal of Orthopsychiatry 19*, 416–426.

Kazadin, A.E. (1997) 'Practioner review: Psychosocial treatments for conduct disorder in children.' *Journal of Child Psychology and Psychiatry 38*, 161–178.

Kemenoff, S., Worchel, F., Prevatt, B. and Willson, V. (1995) 'The effects of video feedback in the context of Milan systemic therapy.' *Journal of Family Psychology 9*, 446–450.

Klin, A. (2000) 'Attributing social meaning to ambiguous visual stimuli in higher functioning autism and Asperger syndrome: The social attribution task.' *Journal of Child Psychology and Psychiatry 41*, 831–846.

Klin, A. and Volkmar, F.R. (2000) 'Treatment and intervention guidelines for individuals with Asperger syndrome.' In A. Klin, F.R. Volkmar and S. Sparrow (eds) *Asperger Syndrome.* New York: Guilford Press, pp.340–366.

Klin, A., Volkmar, F.R. and Sparrow, S. (1992) 'Autistic social dysfunctions: some limitations of the theory of mind hypothesis.' *Journal of Child Psychology and Psychiatry 33*, 861–876.

Klin, A., Sparrow, S.S., de Bildt, A. Cicchetti, D.V., Cohen, D.J. and Volkmar, F.R. (1999) 'A normed study of face recognition in autism and related disorders.' *Journal of Autism and Developmental Disorders 29*, 499–508.

Klin, A., Volkmar, F.R. and Sparrow, S. (2000) *Asperger Syndrome.* New York: Guilford Press.

Klin, A., Jones, W., Schultz, R. and Volkmar, F.R. (2004) 'The enactive mind, or from actions to cognition.' In U. Frith and E. Hill (eds) *Autism: Mind and Brain.* Oxford: Oxford University Press, pp.127–157.

Koning, C. and Magill-Evans, J. (2001) 'Social and language skills in adolescent boys with Asperger syndrome.' *Autism 5*, 23–36.

Korvatska, E., Van de Water, J., Anders, T.F. and Gershwin, M.E. (2002) 'Genetic and immunologic considerations in Autism.' *Neurobiology of Disease 9*, 107–125.

Ladd, G.W. (1984) 'Social skill training with children: Issues in research and practice.' *Clinical Psychology Review 4*, 317–337.

Landa, R. (2000) 'Social language use in Asperger syndrome and high functioning autism.' In A. Klin, F.R. Volkmar and S. Sparrow (eds) *Asperger Syndrome.* New York: Guilford Press, pp.125–155.

Landa, R., Folstein, S.E., and Isaacs, C. (1991) 'Spontaneous narrative-discourse performance of parents of autistic children.' *Journal of Speech and Hearing Research 34*, 1339–1345.

Landa, R., Piven, J., Wzorek, M.M., Gayle, J.O., Chase, G.A. and Folstein, S.E. (1992) 'Social language use in parents of autistic individuals.' *Psychological Medicine 22*, 245–254.

Lapidus, D. (1985) *Developing Communication and Language Skills in Autism.* New York: Nassau Center for Developmental Disabilities.

Lawlor, M., Harpur, J. and James, D. (2004) *Bullying of Asperger Syndrome Adolescents: A Comparison with Typical Peers in Irish Second Level Education.* Navan: Child and Adolescent Mental Health Services.

Lawson, W. (2003) *Build Your Own Life: A Self-Help Guide for Individuals with Asperger Syndrome.* London: Jessica Kingsley Publishers.

Ledgin, N. (2002) *Asperger's and Self-Esteem: Insight and Hope through Famous Role Models.* Arlington, TX: Future Horizons.

LeDoux, J. (2002) *Synaptic Self.* New York: Penguin.

Leslie, A.M. (1994) 'Pretending and believing: Issues in the theory of ToMM.' *Cognition 50*, 211–238.

Long, B. and Schenk, S. (2002) *The Digital Filmmaking Handbook,* 2nd edn. Clifton Park, NY: Charles River Media.

Lord, C. and Paul, R. (1997) 'Language and communication in autism.' In D.J. Cohen and F.R. Volkmar (eds) *Handbook of Autism and Developmental Disorders.* New York: Wiley, pp.195–225.

Marcus, L.L., Kunce, L.J. and Schopler, E. (1997) Working with families. In D.J. Cohen, and F.R. Volkmar (eds) *Handbook of Autism and Pervasive Developmental Disorders.* New York: Wiley, pp. 631–649.

Martin, I. and McDonald, S. (2003) 'Weak coherence, no theory of mind, or executive dysfunction? Solving the puzzle of pragmatic language disorders.' *Brain & Language 85,* 451–466.

Martin, I. and McDonald, S. (2004) 'An exploration of causes of non-literal language problems in individuals with Asperger syndrome.' *Journal of Autism and Developmental Disorders 34,* 311–328.

Mesibov, G.B., Shea, V. and Adams, L.W. (2001) *Understanding Asperger Syndrome and High Functioning Autism.* New York: Kluwer.

Mobbs Henry, F., Reed, V.A. and McAlister, L.L. (1995) 'Adolescents' perceptions of the relative importance of selected communication skills in their positive peer relationships.' *Language, Speech and Hearing Service in Schools 26,* 263–272.

Molloy, H. and Latika, V. (2004) *Asperger Syndrome, Adolescence, and Identity: Looking Beyond the Label.* London: Jessica Kingsley Publishers.

Moyes, R., (2001) *Incorporating Social Goals in the Classroom: A Guide for Teachers and Parents of Children with High-Functioning Autism and Asperger Syndrome.* London: Jessica Kingsley Publishers.

Muhle, R., Trentacoste, S.V. and Rapin, I. (2004) 'The genetics of autism.' *Pediatrics 113,* e472–e486.

Murphy, J.T. (1999) 'Common factors of school-based change.' In M.A. Hubble, B.L. Duncan and S.C. Miller (eds) *The Heart and Soul of Change: What Works in Therapy.* Washington, DC: American Psychological Association, pp.361–386.

Myles, B.S. (2001) 'Understanding the hidden curriculum: An essential social skill for children and youth with Asperger syndrome.' *Intervention in School and Clinic 36,* 279–286.

Myles, B.S. and Adreon, D. (2001) *Asperger Syndrome and Adolescence: Practical Solutions for School Success.* Mission, KS: Autism Asperger Publishing Company.

National Research Council (2001) 'Educating children with autism.' In C. Lord and J. McGee (eds) *Committee on Educational Interventions for Children with Autism.* Washington, DC: National Academy Press.

Nichols, S. and Stich, S.P. (2003) *Mindreading.* Oxford: Oxford University Press.

Nordin, V. and Gillberg, C. (1998) 'The long-term course of autistic disorders: Update on follow-up studies.' *Acta Psychiatrica Scandinavia 97,* 99–108.

Norman, D.A. and Shallice, T. (1986) 'Attention to action: Willed and automatic control of behaviour.' In G.E. Schwartz and D. Shapir (eds) *Consciousness and Self-Regulation.* New York: Plenum Press, pp.1–18.

O'Hanrahan, S. and Fitzgerald, M. (1999) 'Personality traits in parents of people with Autism.' *Irish Journal of Psychological Medicine 16,* 59–60.

Ozonoff, S. and Miller, J.N. (1995) 'Teaching theory of mind: A new approach to social skills training for individuals with autism.' *Journal of Autism and Development Disorders 25,* 415–433.

Ozonoff, S. and Miller, J.N. (1996) 'An exploration of right-hemisphere contributions to the pragmatic impairments of autism.' *Brain and Language 52,* 411–434.

Ozonoff, S. and Pennington, B. (1991) 'Executive functioning deficits in high functioning autistic individuals: Relationship to theory of mind.' *Journal of Child Psychology and Psychiatry 32,* 1081–1105.

Ozonoff, S., Dawson, G. and McPartland, J. (2002) *A Parent's Guide to Asperger Syndrome and High Functioning Autism: How to Meet the Challenges and Help Your Child Thrive.* New York: Guilford Press.

Parisse, C. (1999) 'Cognition and language acquisition in normal and autistic children.' *Journal of Neurolinguistics 12,* 247–269.

Perner, J. (1998) 'The meta-intentional nature of executive functions and theory of mind.' In P. Carruthers and J. Boucher (eds) *Language and Thought: Inderdisciplinary Themes.* Cambridge: Cambridge University Press, pp.270–316.

Perner, J. and Lang, B. (2000) 'Theory of mind and executive function: Is there a developmental relationship?' In S. Baron-Cohen, H. Tager-Flusberg and D.J. Cohen (eds) *Understanding Other Minds: Perspectives from Developmental Cognitive Neuroscience.* Oxford: Oxford University Press, pp.150–181.

Phelps-Teraski, D. and Phelps-Gunn, T. (1992) *Test of Pragmatic Language.* Austin, TX: Pro-Ed.

Piven, J., Chase, G.A., Landa, R., Wzorek, M., Gayle, J., Cloud, D. and Folstein, S. (1991) 'Psychiatric disorders in the parents of autistic individuals.' *Journal of the American Academy of Child and Adolescent Psychiatry 30,* 471.

Premack, D. and Woodruff, G. (1978) 'Does the chimpanzee have a "theory of mind"?' *Behavioural and Brain Sciences 4,* 515–526.

Prizant, B.M., Schuler, A.L. and Wetherby, A.M. (1997) 'Enhancing language and communication development: Language approaches.' In D.J. Cohen and F. Volkmar (eds) *Autism and Pervasive Developmental Disorders.* New York: Wiley, pp.572–605.

Rinaldi, W. (1992) *The Social Use of Language Programme: Enhancing the Social Communication of Children and Teenagers with Special Educational Needs.* Windsor: NFER-Nelson.

Rinaldi, W. (2001) *Language Difficulties in an Educational Context.* London: Whurr Publishers.

Robertson, I. (2000) *Mind Sculpture: Unleashing your Brain's Potential.* New York: Bantam Press.

Rogers, S.J. (2000) 'Interventions that facilitate socialization in children with autism.' *Journal of Autism and Development Disorders 30,* 399–409.

Rubenstein, J.L.R. and Merzenich, M.M. (2003) 'Model of autism: Increased ratio of excitation/inhibition in key neural systems.' *Genes, Brain and Behaviour 2,* 255–267.

Russell, A.J., Mataix-Cols, D., Anson, M. and Murphy, D.G.M. (2005) 'Obsessions and compulsions in Asperger syndrome and high-functioning autism.' *British Journal of Psychiatry 186,* 525–528.

Santangelo, S.L. and Tsatsanis, K. (2005) 'What is known about autism: Genes, brain and behavior.' *American Journal of Pharmacogenomics 5,* 71–92.

Savidge, C., Christie, D., Brooks, E., Stein, S.M. and Wolpert, M. (2004) 'A pilot social skills group for socially disorganized children.' *Clinical Child Psychology and Psychiatry 9,* 289–296.

Schopler, E. and Mesibov, G.B. (eds) (1998) *Asperger Syndrome or High Functioning Autism?* New York: Kluwer.

Schultz, R.T., Gauthier, I., Klin, A., Fulbright, R.K., Anderson, A.W., Volkmar, F.R., Skudlarski, P., Lacadie, C., Cohen, D.J. and Gore, J.C. (2000) 'Abnormal ventral temporal cortical activity during face discrimination among individuals with autism and Asperger syndrome.' *Archives of General Psychiatry 57,* 331–340.

SDQINFO (2005) www.sdqinfo.com (accessed July 2005).

Searle, J. (1975) 'Indirect speech acts.' In P. Cole and J. Morgan, (eds) *Syntax and Semantics, Vol. 3, Speech Acts.* New York: Academic Press, pp.59–82.

Sergeant, J.A., Geurts, H., Huijbregts, S., Scheres, A. and Oosterlaan, J. (2003) 'The top and the bottom of ADHD: A neuropsychological perspective.' *Neuroscience & Biobehavioral Reviews 27,* 583–592.

Shore, S. (2003) *Beyond the Wall: Personal Experiences with Autism and Asperger Syndrome,* 2nd edn. Shawnee Mission, KS: Autism Asperger Publishing Company.

Shriberg, L.D., Paul, R., McSweeny, J.L., Klin, A., Cohen, D.J. and Volkmar, F.R. (2001) 'Speech and prosody characteristics of adolescents and adults with high-functioning autism and Asperger syndrome.' *Journal of Speech, Language, and Hearing Research, 44,* 1097–1115.

Sirota, K.G. (2004) 'Positive politeness as discourse process: Politeness practices of high-functioning children with autism and Asperger syndrome.' *Discourse Studies 6,* 229–251.

Slater-Walker, G. and Slater-Walker, C. (2002) *An Asperger Marriage.* London: Jessica Kingsley Publishers.

Smith, S.C. and Pennells, S.M. (1993) 'Bereaved children and adolescents.' In K. Nath Dwivedi (ed) *Group Work with Children and Adolescents: A Handbook.* London: Jessica Kingsley Publishers, pp.195–208.

Sparrow, S.S., Balla, D. and Cicchetti, D.V. (1984) *Vineland Adaptive Behaviour Scales*. Circle Pines, MN: American Guidance Service Publishing.

Spence, S.H. (2003) 'Social skills training with children and young people: Theory, evidence and practice.' *Child and Adolescent Mental Health 8*, 84–96.

Sperber, D. and Wilson, D. (1995) *Relevance: Communication and Cognition*, 2nd edn. Oxford: Blackwell.

Stephenson, C. (1993) 'Use of drama.' In K. Nath Dwivedi (ed) *Group Work with Children and Adolescents*. London: Jessica Kingsley Publishers, pp.170–182.

Sturm, H., Fernell, E. and Gillberg, C. (2004) 'Autism spectrum disorders in children with normal intellectual levels: Associated impairments and subgroups.' *Developmental Medicine And Child Neurology 46*, 444–447.

Szatmari, P., Bartolucci, G. and Bremner, R. (1989) 'Asperger's syndrome and autism: Comparisons on early history and outcome.' *Developmental Medicine and Child Neurology 31*, 253–279.

Tager-Flusberg, H. (1995) 'Dissociation in form and function in the acquisition of language by autistic children.' In H. Tager-Flusberg (ed) *Constraints on Language Acquisition: Studies of Atypical Children*. Hillsdale, NJ: Lawrence Erlbaum, pp.175–194.

Tantam, D. (2000) 'Adolescenc and adulthood of individuals with Asperger syndrome.' In A. Klin, F.R. Volkmar and S. Sparrow (eds) *Asperger Syndrome*. New York: Guilford Press, pp.369–399.

Trillingsgaard, A. (1999) 'The script model in relation to autism.' *European Journal of Child and Adolescent Psychiatry 8*, 45–49.

Troia, G.A. and Whitney, S.D. (2003) 'A close look at the efficacy of Fast ForWord Language for children with academic weaknesses.' *Contemporary Educational Psychology 28*, 465–494.

Valdizan, J.R., Zarazaga-Andia, I., Abril-Villalba, B., Sans-Capdevila, O. and Mendez-Garcia, M. (2003) 'Face recognition in autism.' *Revista de Neurologia 36* 1186–1189.

Vaughn, S. and Lancelotta, G.X. (1990) 'Teaching interpersonal social skills to poorly accepted students: Peer-pairing versus non-peer-pairing.' *Journal of School Psychology 28*, 181–188.

Webb, B.J., Miller, S.P., Pierce, T.B., Strawser, S. and Jones, W.P. (2004) 'Effects of social skill instruction for high-functioning adolescents with autism spectrum disorders.' *Focus on Autism and Other Developmental Disabilities 19*, 53–62.

Welchew, D.E., Ashwin, C., Berkouk, K., Salvador, R., Suckling, J., Baron-Cohen, S. and Bullmore, E. (2005) 'Functional disconnectivity of the medial temporal lobe in Asperger's syndrome.' *Biological Psychiatry 57*, 991–998.

Weschler, D. (1992) *Manual for the Weschler Intelligence Scale for Children*, 3rd edn. San Antonio, TX: Psychological Corporation.

Weston, J. (1996) *Directing Actors*. Studio City, CA: Michael Weise Publications.

Whang, P.L., Fawcett, S.B. and Mathews, R.M. (1984) 'Teaching job-related social skills to learning disabled adolescents.' *Analysis and Intervention in Developmental Disabilities 4*, 29–38.

Whitehill, M.B., Hersen, M. and Bellack, A.S. (1980) 'Conversation skills training for socially isolated children.' *Behaviour Research and Therapy 18*, 217–225.

Wiig, E.H. and Secord, W. (1989) *Test of Language Competence – Expanded*. San Antonio, TX: Psychological Corporation.

Wing, L. (1981) 'Asperger syndrome: A clinical account.' *Psychological Medicine 19*, 115–130.

Wing, L. and Gould, J. (1979) 'Severe impairments of social interaction and associated abnormalities in children: Epidemiology and classification.' *Journal of Autism and Childhood Schizophrenia 9*, 11–29.

World Health Organisation (1990) *International Classification of Diseases: Tenth Revision*. Geneva: WHO.

Yoshida, Y. and Uchiyama, T. (2004) 'The clinical necessity for assessing attention deficit/hyperactivity disorder (AD/HD) symptoms in children with high-functioning pervasive developmental disorder (PDD)'. *European Child & Adolescent Psychiatry 13*, 307–314.

Yovel, G. and Kanwisher, N. (2004) 'Face perception: Domain specific, not process specific.' *Neuron 44*, 889–898.

Subject Index

Page numbers in *italics* indicate figures, tables or boxes.

Author Index

Page numbers in *italics* indicate tables.